GIVE ME STRENGTH

Strength and Conditioning Training for Seniors Over 60

Fight Aging Using Simple At-Home Workouts to Get Stronger, Improve Balance and Increase Energy

100+ Exercises and Workouts

By Matthew Case

Published by SMC Media LLC

Table of Contents

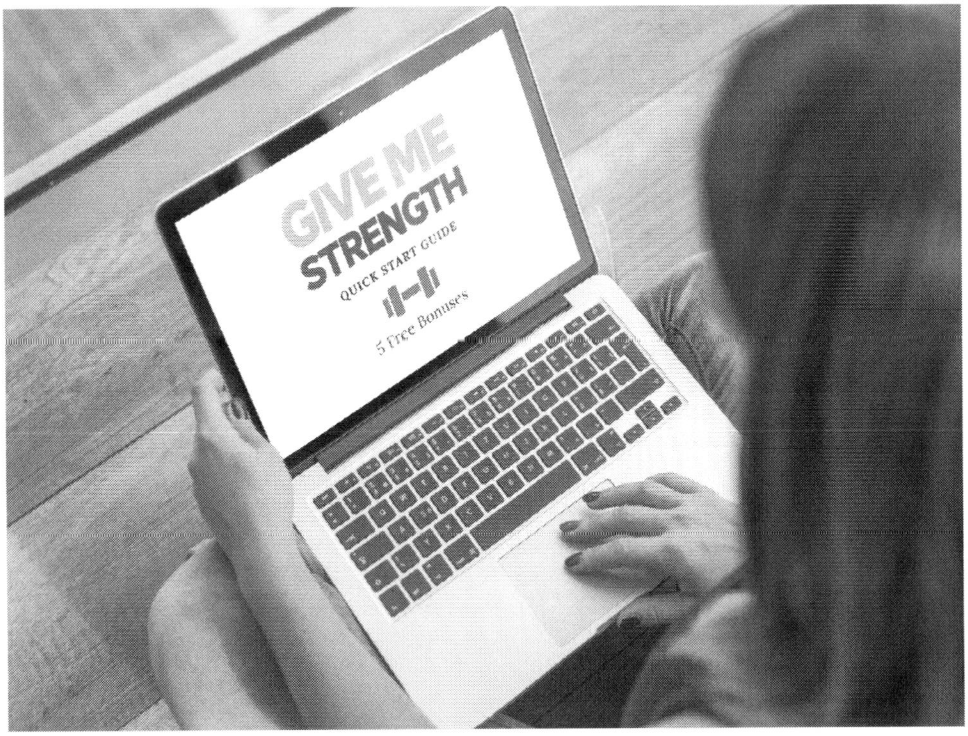

A FREE GIFT TO OUR READERS!

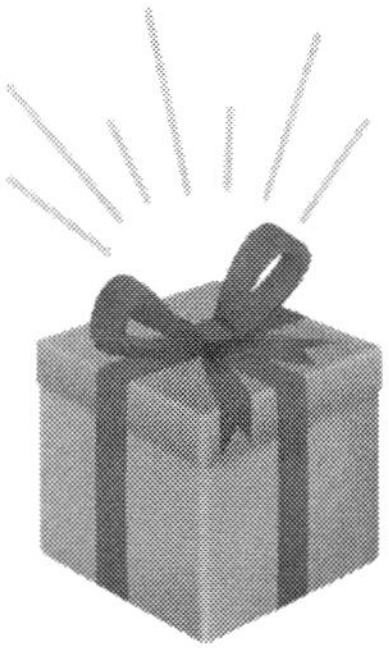

Before you begin this book, please take advantage of the **5 Free Bonuses** from the **Give Me Strength Quick Start Guide**. Inside this guide, you will receive:

Free Bonus #1 - Dancing for Strength Bonus Workout

In this bonus workout, you'll see additional core and balance exercises and a special "Dancing for Strength" workout. It will feature a weblink to a custom music playlist to give you additional "pep in your step" while you exercise.

Free Bonus #2 - 5x5 Fitness Challenge

This incredible freebie will provide you with a quick roadmap for establishing motivation, goals, better sleep, and much more. I encourage…no, I challenge you to complete this 5x5 Fitness Challenge. Complete 1 challenge per day for a total of 5 in 5 days! See Free Bonus #3 for the companion piece to this.

Free Bonus #3 - Transformation Tools

These worksheets, or tools rather, are useful for the 5x5 Fitness Challenge. They include; find your 5 whys, 5 fitness goals, 5 ways to better sleep, 5 hints to stay hydrated, and 5 tips to improve your thought life. They are easy to print, use and even share with others.

Free Bonus #4 - Workout Calendar

This fantastic freebie is a calendar template that you can use to track your workouts during the month. It's easy to get off track, but this calendar will help you avoid this by helping you plan the month and showcase all the hard work you've done!

Free Bonus #5 - Give Me Strength Recipes, Shopping List

This bonus provides three yummy recipes for a fitness lifestyle. It also contains a shopping list and will offer healthy suggestions for grocery shopping. Good nutrition is key to successful strength and conditioning training.

To receive your 5 free bonuses, scan this QR code:

Introduction

"If I knew I was going to live this long, I would have taken better care of myself!"

– George Burns.

These words are a confession of a senior (a world-famous actor and comedian) who lived to be 100 years old. His sentiments are felt by many all over the world.

It's no secret that by age 60, most become consumed by negative thoughts of fragility, loss of independence, and risk of fall-related injuries. In addition, years of sedentary behavior leading to weight gain, loss of muscles, and body aches and pains, have many seniors worried about their futures. And rightfully so, because the surprising findings of a new study reveal that skipping out on exercise is one of the worst things you can do to your health.

Lack of exercise is deadlier than smoking, diabetes, heart disease, and high blood pressure. A study done by Cleveland Clinic Foundation on more than 122,000 seniors over 23 years revealed that inactivity increases your chances of premature death more than hypertension, cholesterol, or drinking.

The study tracked the participants to determine the link between inactivity and mortality. The comparison between the seniors that scored the highest and those that scored lowest on a treadmill stress test showed that the least fit of the bunch had a 500% increased chance of dying prematurely than the fittest group.

So comparatively, if a smoker is only 1.4 times more likely to die prematurely than the average person and a diabetic person is 1.3 times more likely to die prematurely, you are five times more likely to die from a sedentary lifestyle. How alarming are these findings? Are you sitting up yet?

Still, many seniors wait until they are stiff, sore, discouraged, beat down, and falling apart at the seams to do something about their health. The big question is…

Why?

Some feel too sick, too tired, or too old to exercise. Others feel too out-of-shape to start (or have other health issues) and have given up. Others associate old age with being feeble and have resolved to be sedentary. They assume and associate loss of balance, weakness, and general inactivity with old age – an inevitable process that no man can escape. They're wrong.

More and more research indicates symptoms such as loss of balance are manifestations of long-term inactivity and not age. But, conversely, physical activity, be it endurance, balance, strength, or flexibility, will add extra years to your life. And one of the essential variables we'll explore in this book is the critical need for strength and conditioning training (to increase muscle mass).

Muscle mass significantly declines with age. You lose approximately 3-5% of muscle mass every decade beginning from the fourth. From 50, you lose 1-2% of muscle mass every year. Think about that. Our muscles are a crucial contributor to bone strength and balance. They keep you strong, help burn calories, improve heart health, and reduce your risk of injury.

Without stronger muscles, your mobility and independence are at considerable risk.

Mom's Health Journey

While talking about the fantastic benefits of exercise and strength training, I will briefly introduce you to my mom and share her incredible journey towards recovery. In the late summer of 2018, my mom, Nancy, whom I love dearly, was preparing to sell her big house to downsize. She had lately begun to struggle with back and leg pain, but the rigors of the big move exacerbated it significantly, and the discomfort in her lower back started to magnify even more. Nevertheless, due to the need to relocate, she forged on ahead through the pain as she moved into her new home.

By the time her move was over, the pain was severe; she was walking crooked and bent over – honestly, she could barely walk a half block or stand in place. By 2019, her quality of life diminished as the pain gradually increased to where she sought consultation with her GP, a neurologist, neurosurgeon, and spine surgeon—including a second opinion at an internationally well-known health institution. After numerous tests, all consults recommended physical therapy, Rx, spinal injections, and back surgery. While physical therapy helped some, the other recommendations scared her, so she searched for holistic/natural alternatives.

She extensively researched diets, nutrition, supplements, and exercises and started implementing what made sense. She joined an online fitness program and began regular strength training exercises, movement routines, yoga, stretches, acupuncture, and chiropractic care (including spinal decompression treatments). Her health began to improve significantly following this. She lost weight, slept better, walked much longer distances, and could stand in place with a straight back. She is convinced that regular strength training exercise, movement, and nutrition have improved her energy and quality of life. She continues with this new active lifestyle and is in excellent health today.

As my mom's story emphasizes, no one can halt the proverbial ticking of the clock, but she and many others have proven that you have the power to slow the process...and live better!

Strength training improves that possibility even as we age. It helps us preserve a healthy weight and can even help manage, if not prevent, conditions like arthritis, high blood pressure, and heart disease, among other maladies. Yet, sadly, strength training is often overlooked.

Most people don't understand that strength training is as crucial as aerobics or other exercises. Aerobic exercise certainly has numerous cardiovascular benefits that can add valuable years to your life. But strength training ensures that these additional years are rewarding and full of energy and vigor.

In this book, a unique manual written after years of experience, I will show you a clear and safe strategy for proper strength and fitness training. You will receive persuasive reasons (including scientific data) on "why" you should apply these strategies to your life…without delay. Finally, I will show you why strength and conditioning training is the missing piece of the puzzle: the piece that conditions your muscles and gives them power and agility so you can stay fit, active, and independent in your senior years.

My love for fitness and health runs deep. As the son of a teacher and a coach, I fell in love with higher education and athletics at a young age. I worked with elite athletes and coached at many different levels. While attending Northwestern University, I became an All-American wrestler, team captain, and recipient of the Big Ten Medal of Honor. And after graduation, I trained for Olympic and World Championship teams.

So, I have been a fitness enthusiast all my life. But my mom, who is on her recovery journey, has been the biggest inspiration behind this book. Her story is one of hope, which is the message I want to give you. I know that better nutrition and strength and conditioning workouts can help you prepare for and recover from injuries and ailments that will eventually surface in your life if they haven't already.

I want everyone to be mentally equipped and physically prepared as we cross into the golden years of our lives. My own goal is to stay healthy and fit to allow me to give more of myself to my wife and children as I age. What are your goals? What is your motivation? I'd love you to join me on this journey and figure that out together.

This book seeks to answer one central question, "*How can you reclaim your health, balance, strength, agility, and vitality and maintain a healthy weight through strength training and conditioning?*"

What if I showed you some expert-vetted, field-tested, science-based approaches proven to build strength, balance, power, and stretching abilities? What if I gave you tips and strategies to avoid injuries, chart your progress, and keep your workout sessions fun, active and exciting? What if I showed you how to tone your body, fortify your bones, strengthen your muscles, build a robust and injury-proof body, and add confidence to your life?

This book doesn't claim to have the answers to lasting youth. Instead, it illuminates a few key strength and conditioning strategies that help you rebuild and improve overall strength. This book is the apex of my personal experiences and my mother's. It's my eye-to-eye interaction with elite athletes I have trained alongside, coached, and helped overcome challenges and setbacks. And it's what my mom has learned along the way in her recovery. It's also a collection of persuasive reasons (using scientific data) why you need to build muscle. Finally, it will reveal some great studies in strength and conditioning.

All is not lost. You can rebuild and reconstruct the broken pieces to create a stronger, better balanced, more energetic version of yourself. Yes, you can do it! And I will teach you how in this book.

Let's get started!

Chapter 1
Give Me Strength:
The What and The Why

"The afternoon knows what the morning never suspected."

- Robert Frost

OUR BODIES WHEN WE AGE

So, you are officially "out of your prime"? What's next?

A-list Hollywood actors and actresses aside, wrinkles and gray hair will slowly catch up with us all. And it's usually inevitable that we will lose some (if not all) of those thick-flowing lustrous youthful locks we once had. Sorry, Fabio. But there is no big surprise here. What is surprising is that most of us have no idea how aging affects the totality of our sexuality, bones, muscles, or brain. If we did, I think we'd all probably pay a bit closer attention. Keep reading, and you'll see what I mean.

As a starting point, our cells' basic structures, processes, and functionality change over time. And while our bodies make over 200 different cells, these cells act somewhat similarly as we age. So when all of these different kinds of cells start to get older, the weakening of our organs and tissues follow hand in hand, consequently leading to the declining performance of our body's systems.

As our internal systems decline, various things happen that reveal the physical effects of aging. For one, the outer skin layers of our bodies can start to become thinner, fragile, translucent, and inelastic. These occurrences are often because of the declining quality of the protein in our bodies called collagen. Collagen strengthens our skin, joints, hair, and many other amazing things.

In addition to collagen depletion and its effects on the skin, hair, and joints, other things like our teeth, hearing, eyes, sexuality, and even taste buds take a hit. For example, research has shown that we might lose half of our taste buds by age 60. This loss can lead to an unhealthy diet to compensate for our flavor loss and produce extra weight as our metabolism loses steam.

Additional studies show that we may lose muscle mass as early as our 30s – both men and women. The muscles lost are replaced by fat, so by the time they hit 75, the average person's body fat percentage will be twice as much as in their 20s. As the muscles lose strength, flexibility, and stability, our balance quickly jumps on the same bandwagon.

And yes, we can shrink too. So no, it's not just a figment of your imagination. An article published by *The Wallstreet Journal* states that after 40, we shrink a quarter to a third of an inch every decade. So the loss of our height can be firmly attributed to our muscle mass loss and declining bone health.

Oh, and I almost forget (hehe) that our brains start slipping with age too, most notably, the parts of our brain responsible for learning, movement, and planning. These reside respectively in the frontal lobe, hippocampus, and cerebellum. Even though our big 3-pound brains have roughly 100 billion neurons, we still begin losing around 50,000 neurons every day after the 30th decade. But there's good news! Studies have shown that despite the natural aging process, our brains still adapt well to this loss of cells. Like the body, the mind can be strengthened and conditioned too using various word games, memorization techniques, puzzles, etc. In addition, the last twenty years of research on the brain have shown how much the mind can balance itself as it loses effectiveness in other areas. This research proves that our aging bodies are still highly adaptable.

All told, gerontologists believe that aging could be somewhat counterintuitive. Believe it or not, we generally get happier and more content as we approach our senior years. Life is more of a U-shaped curve. We are more joyful as kids, a feeling which diminishes as we go into our adult years -think quarter-life and midlife crises, and things begin to look up again in our senior years.

And the good news doesn't end there. New research shows that while the aging process is inevitable, there is much we can do to slow down the process, increase our productivity as we age, maintain an active life, spend more time with our loved ones and focus on things we enjoy.

Old myths have always associated aging with loss of functionality in different body systems and, consequently, a point of view on life that becomes depressing. But, new research shows that lifestyle choices can significantly impact aging mentally and physically. Furthermore, those choices have the power to either keep the aging status quo, accelerate it or slow it down. So, we can do a lot to stop and reverse the aging process. The choice is up to us!

WHY DO WE NEED TO EXERCISE?

Our bodies are built for movement. They were designed to lift, walk, push and pull. A few centuries back, people engaged in vigorous physical activities for survival; they had to work hard just to acquire, nay…capture something to eat. With the advent of turn of century technology, we have dramatically reduced our regular physical work and movement. We drive to work or work from our comfy homes, sit at our desks for hours, and then come home to watch our favorite movies and T.V. shows. If we're retired, we have everything we need, from door-to-door grocery delivery to having our favorite restaurant deliver us any meal, even snacks! It sounds like a great life, right? I mean, everything is right where we need it. These benefits can be pretty fantastic and offer us an excellent, uncomplicated life. I've personally taken advantage of many of these conveniences.

Despite the pros of the "easy life," it often creates a passive mindset, exacerbating our aging and kicking it into high gear. It forms a big gap between what our bodies naturally need and what we do daily. What's exciting, however, is that something unique can help bridge this gap and move us out of this sedentary meets aging conundrum.

One significant lifestyle choice will make a magnificent difference in helping our bodies achieve what they truly need. It is…are you ready for it, drum roll please…did you guess it? That's right, it's exercise. Yes, exercise is one of the best lifestyle choices you can make that can hyper speed us into what our bodies need or are craving. If you don't believe me, ask your body after a few weeks of consistently using this book.

The decision to and the act of exercise helps us combat and have victory in the aging process...period. What's equally exciting is that we have the power to make that decision for ourselves. By reading this book, you have already made a massive step in the right direction. Choosing effective and consistent exercise routines can significantly delay many health and aging-related issues. In addition, exercise can help us keep chronic illnesses at bay and almost magically make many of our aches and pains disappear. In short, our ailments don't have to interfere with the full enjoyment of life at the top of the aforementioned U-shaped curve. We just need to decide.

So what are some aging issues that can potentially keep us from enjoying the rest of our lives? And how can exercise help? So let's digress for a minute and let some of the newest data sink into our heads.

Studies have shown that over 650,000 people in the U.S. die from heart disease yearly. It's the primary cause of death in American men and kills one in every four. Heart disease is also the leading cause of death in the U.S., not just in men but in almost every demographic.

Another thing science is discovering is that proper exercise and nutrition reduce cardiac risks such as obesity, high cholesterol, and high blood pressure, which has an impressive preventative influence on congestive heart failure. A Harvard Alumni Study supports the theory, which found that exercise reduced active seniors' risk of heart attack by up to 39% compared to inactive peers. This observation was mind-blowing, and multiple studies have backed this up.

Atherosclerosis (narrowing of arteries due to fat and cholesterol accumulation) usually causes stroke, the third leading cause of death in the U.S. Stroke and heart disease have so much in common, especially regarding the risk factors. For this reason, it makes sense when the same study concluded that exercise reduces the risk of stroke. The Harvard Alumni Study reported a 24% reduction in heart disease when participants did mild exercises and an even better 46% reduced risk when the activity was moderate or intensive.

Cancer might not be so straightforward, but multiple studies show that exercise could help fight it off to a certain extent. One excellent example is colon cancer. According to a follow-up study by Harvard Health Professionals, the risk of developing colon cancer is reduced by up to 47% in highly active males. While these findings are not entirely conclusive, many studies also rally behind the idea of reduced risk of prostate cancer in active seniors.

So as recent studies are proving, exercise can be essential for preventing heart disease, stroke, and cancer. Even better, there is proof that exercise can reduce the risk of many disabling and stressful conditions such as hypertension, prostatic hyperplasia, osteoporosis, diabetes, and gallbladder attacks, among others. If these aren't convincing enough, you might be impressed that the study showed that physical activity could reduce the risk of impotence in senior men by up to 30%. Men, are you listening?

The point here is that we are more likely to live longer, healthier, productive lives and slow the aging process if we make exercise part of our lives. According to multiple studies, we add around two hours of life expectancy for every hour of physical activity. These hours add up to two years over our lives, but only if the exercise is regular.

Fortunately, it's never too late to start, as reported by a mortality analysis done at Harvard University. There was a 24% reduced death rate in sedentary men who started regular physical activity at age 45 compared to men who remained inactive all their lives. Even when they became active later in life, previously sedentary people gained up to 1.6 years in life expectancy. Other studies from England and Norway back up the findings of this research.

So after reading about the data, can we at least agree that using our bodies keeps them fit, youthful, and younger? The evidence is there. If so, let's keep going to explore more specifically what we need to do. It's one thing to know exercise has fantastic rewards, and it's quite another to understand how to reap those rewards. But this is why we are here, to explore the whys and the hows together. For our framework, we must first start to develop a balanced, holistic exercise program that incorporates the following;

Resistance

Resistance builds muscle mass, making you stronger and more energetic. It's the key to the preservation of bone calcium as we age. You may need an instructor to learn the basics, but proper home programs work efficiently.

Endurance

Improving your endurance has the best effect on cardiovascular function. Endurance exercises have proven benefits such as reduced heart rate, flexible arteries, improved working performance, and maintenance of heart muscle strength. In addition, endurance improves our metabolism, which generally slows down with age while reducing body fat. Finally, we may struggle with sleep in our senior years, but better endurance can improve it and reduce anxiety, depression, and stress.

Balance

So you want to slow down the aging process? Balance exercises will help you with that. It's the trick to aging gracefully, and staying clear of fractures, falls, and injuries that lead to crippling disabilities and pain.

Flexibility

Flexibility training keeps us agile. Stretching is key to part of the preparation process and during the cool-down process of exercise. Yoga also has terrific flexibility techniques, many of which can be used as a warm-up before resistance and endurance training.

WHAT IS STRENGTH AND CONDITIONING (S&C) TRAINING?

At its core, strength and conditioning training is any movement-based exercise program that makes you stronger and builds better endurance. As the name suggests, strength and conditioning training improves our muscles' endurance, power, and size. Effectual strength and conditioning incorporates resistance (for strength), cardiovascular techniques (for endurance), and core and stretching (for balance and flexibility).

In the past, many people have associated S&C training with things like Olympic powerlifting or professional football hill sprint drills that only elite athletes can manage. Still, the newest data shows that is a complete misnomer. While these exercises are certainly part of strength and condition training for high-performance athletes, simple resistance bands, lightweight dumbbells, and body weight exercises are equally effective in providing the resistance and endurance we need. Moreover, the same principles used with elite athletes transcend into workouts and exercises for us, right in the convenience of our homes.

WHY IS S&C IMPORTANT

More and more people are embracing S&C training as additional evidence-based research is being revealed to us, especially now that more are personally experiencing the benefits. People are no longer looking at S&C training as a niche for high-performance athletes and bodybuilders. Depending on your individual needs, you can choose tailor-made S&C exercises (available in this book) that focus on qualities such as agility or mobility, endurance or flexibility, pain management, and core stability. S&C training is adaptable.

One incredible benefit of S&C training is injury prevention. By developing better movements, strength and conditioning training can help seniors improve balance and proprioception (perception and awareness of one's body) to reduce the risk of falling and related injuries. Recent studies have also shown that S&C increases the functionality and durability of our muscles, bones, joints, ligaments, and tendons, so if we fall, these areas of our bodies can more quickly adapt and recover from injuries and fractures.

S&C training also helps minimize the effect of bone loss as we age. For instance, our bones are perpetually evolving, and we get newer bone created after our bodies break down our older bone tissue. Research shows that our bodies build newer bones quicker than destroying older bones in our younger years. As a result, our bone mass gradually improves and reaches its peak performance at around age 30. After 30, however, our bones still grow, but we slowly start losing bone mass.

The rate at which we develop weak and brittle bones, also known as osteoporosis, will be determined by how much bone mass we've acquired by age 30. The more bone mass we accumulate, the more bone reserve we'll have left later in life. So the sooner we can pack on more bone density, the better our chances are of keeping osteoporosis at bay.

And as we replace fat with muscle (yet another result of S&C training), our posture improves. In addition, our circulation and respiratory systems, which rely heavily on balance and posture, receive help. And last but not least, we start to look and feel much better, which boosts our self-confidence.

So as you can see, there is so much more to S&C than just high-intensity weight lifting, powerlifting, and bodybuilding categories. S&C exercises can truly transform anyone's body, health, physical performance, confidence, and consequently, our lives regardless of the fitness category to which we aspire.

What is the "conditioning" part of S&C training, and why is it important?

While we shouldn't get too technical here, it's essential to distinguish between strength training and the conditioning part of the training process. Combined with strength training, conditioning adds a cardiovascular component to training, offering several benefits.

1. It improves heart health. As our heart works to pump blood during conditioning, it opens the blood vessels and maintains their flexibility. As a result, our blood pressure and risk of stroke are reduced.
2. It helps burn more calories, which kicks our metabolism into a higher gear.
3. It also adds more endurance to our muscles which will help us get less tired while exercising.
4. It works our muscles, so they are more powerful.
5. Tones and shapes our bodies.

Conditioning is essentially a form of cardiovascular exercise. It's a way to keep the heart rate up, burn fat, burn calories, and keep our metabolisms churning. Strength training is essentially doing exercises that increase our strength and muscle properties. When strength training is married with conditioning training, they maximize each other's effectiveness. They're a match made in heaven. They complement each other, making the other one even better.

What is resistance training, and why should I know about it?

When you read about different kinds of training, there are many different terms, which can get a little confusing. For example, resistance training is essentially the same thing as strength training. Some use other words to describe the similar process of either weight training, bodyweight training, or resistance band training. And some experts will get into the weeds on the minor differences, but we will use these terms synonymously throughout this book as most scientific studies define them as the same animal.

So, now you know what happens to our bodies as we age, what strength and conditioning training is, and why we all need to make exercise part of daily life. Chapter 2 will explore the benefits of S&C training in detail. These benefits will help keep us mindful as we approach the motivational aspect of our endeavors: getting and staying healthy and fit.

Chapter 2
The Good, The Bad, and The Benefits

"Nature gives you the face you have at twenty, it is up to you to merit the face you have at fifty."

- Coco Chanel

As briefly discussed in the previous chapter, there are benefits to S&C training. We've also learned that scientific data continues to support the advantages of following a disciplined S&C program as time passes. In this chapter, we aim to familiarize ourselves with the irrefutable benefits that can help with our motivation, especially when things get tough. So please stay with me. It's about to get very interesting!

Studies show that the average life expectancy in 1914 was 55 years, compared to 80 years today. Thankfully we now have (on average) an additional 25 years to do stuff! Wouldn't it be amazing if those extra years we have now were active and completely independent? And when I say "independent," I mean not needing the help of a cane, walker, or another person to get around.

Walking without help is one of the most critical determinants of our ability to live independent lives. Other activities that show our independence include things like, bathing, dressing, eating, and getting out of bed without assistance.

When we're healthy, we usually take these "mundane" daily activities for granted. Especially if we've yet to have any significant health issues, however, it is usually not until our health takes an unexpected nosedive that we often long for just enough strength to regain this rudimentary independence. It is then where we look into the mirror (if we can get to a mirror) and say to ourselves, "GIVE ME STRENGTH!"

One study published on Lifestyle Interventions and Independence for Elders (LIFE) concluded that we must start doing something about our health today to prohibit this kind of thing from happening. The study confirmed what we already know. Inactivity is the most substantial contributor to loss of independence and disability in our golden years.

Researchers from the study recommend exercises that build strength and balance as the first step toward minimizing the risk of mobility disability. In the study's conclusion, the researchers echoed suggestions from the United States Physical Activity Guidelines; "*move more, move often.*" This philosophy is certainly a great place to start.

As you might expect and have probably witnessed, sedentary seniors are less likely to live independent lives and do everyday activities without help than their physically active peers. There are no surprises here. But what might surprise you is how quickly we can "move more, and move often" out of a sedentary category and into an "active category" by genuinely understanding and putting into practice the immense benefits of S&C training.

But, before we discuss those exciting benefits, let's briefly explore some of the myths of S&C training and identify what could be potential stumbling blocks towards pursuing a healthier mind and body. And please don't skip over these. They are important. Almost every one of us has some excuse or lie in the back of our heads that casts doubts and stops us from changing our habits, especially as we age.

MYTHS OF STRENGTH TRAINING

Lie 1: Older adults can't get stronger or build muscle.

What if I told you the exact opposite is true? In reality, strength and conditioning training will build muscle and strength despite our age. Multiple studies have proven that we can build muscle and increase physical strength into our nineties.

Lie 2: I'm too old, weak, sick, or frail to start.

This lie is about the "I'll *break my hip/ankle*," "I'll *have a heart attack while working out*," or "*I am in pain, so I'll just avoid it*" kind of excuses. Unless a qualified medical healthcare provider tells you any of these based on a condition you may already have, it's just fear talking.

Pain shouldn't be an excuse either. Because exercise improves flexibility and stability, seniors with arthritis are encouraged by more and more doctors to exercise regularly. Exercise reduces joint stiffness and overall pain, all while reducing fatigue. Motion is lotion!

Lie 3: It's too late to start.

Our bodies benefit from exercise, no matter when we start. You may have been sedentary throughout the years, but you can still add extra years to your life if you start now. Do not delay! The catchphrase "better late than never" has never been more relevant than it is in beginning exercise at an older age. Even if we start later in life, exercise will still reduce our risk of developing diabetes, heart disease, different types of cancer, and high blood pressure.

Lie 4: I would preferably focus on my mind rather than my body.

It's virtually impossible to have one without the other. You are more likely to be in a healthy state of mind if your body is healthy. A recent study published in *Nature Magazine* outlines that exercising, especially with others or in nature, reduces anxiety and depression. In addition, it can slow the onset or reduce the progression of dementia.

Lie 5: Strength and conditioning training is for young people, primarily men.

Strength and conditioning can benefit anyone willing to put in the work. It is just as crucial for women as it is for men. Women lose bone mass every other year after menopause, which makes S&C training even more critical because it helps them slow down bone loss and the onset of osteoporosis.

Lie 6: S&C training is dangerous and too difficult to learn.

Strength and conditioning are as safe as any other exercise when done correctly. It doesn't matter how weak you feel you are; there is an S&C exercise routine that will suit your capability. And you don't have to start with weights if you are not ready; you can begin incrementally and gradually pick up the pace. You'll learn in this book that simple bodyweight exercises will accomplish the mission. This book will also provide tailor-made workouts and ala carte options.

Lie 7: It's impossible to find someone to exercise with at my age.

Choosing an exercise routine and doing it is the most challenging part; finding a workout buddy isn't. But, you can always find someone or inspire someone to start taking good care of their health. Join your local YMCA/WCA, a walking club, or seniors club and see what they offer. Even better if exercise is part of it. It's an excellent opportunity to hang out with people who love and value exercise.

Talk with other seniors about your life and passion; you might be surprised by the number of like-minded people you meet or inspire to start or join the journey. Maybe they were looking for inspiration or someone to work out with, just like you.

Lie 8: It's too expensive and out of reach for me.

You can break the bank for equipment and memberships, but you don't have to. Simply find some comfy shoes and workout clothes and go for a walk. Weed the garden in your backyard for a few hours if you'd like. If the weather outside is terrible, you can even exercise/lift weights using canned foods or water bottles that are effective lightweights. They work well as resistance training equipment. Or simply try walking up and down the stairs several times. Remember, "move more, move often."

Lie 9: I've never done it before; what difference will it make?

A lot. It will make a lot of difference.

If you start now, you can atone for a lifetime of inactivity. Even into our nineties, studies report that we can boost muscle strength and physical fitness through strength and conditioning training. In addition, the same studies report that even if we start later in life, our risk of chronic illnesses or their symptoms can be reduced even if we start exercising later in life. So it's never too late to begin when it comes to exercise.

Lie 10: I don't have enough time.

We all know that we give importance to the things necessary to us. If we can just internalize and grasp the significance of regular exercise, precisely strength and conditioning, then we are on our way to countering this lie. Please keep reading, and we'll help you with this.

We don't need to visit an expensive gym nor spend hours working out to receive benefits from exercise. The most important thing is to start exercising and stick with it. After you see some results, you'll soon see it's worth putting in the time.

KEY BENEFITS OF STRENGTH AND CONDITIONING TRAINING:

1. Strengthens and Builds Lean Muscles

Many of you may remember the old cartoon called Popeye. I watched it a lot as a kid because I was fascinated by Popeye's ability to get instantly stronger. But, as you might surmise, I quickly learned that the spinach I ate didn't exactly work as it did for him. So while we can't tap into those magic cans of spinach (that seemed to appear out of nowhere), we can still achieve real help for our muscles when we need them to be stronger.

As we grow older, we continue to lose muscle mass. Sarcopenia (sar·co·pe·ni·a) is the medical term for progressive muscle loss as we age. Studies reveal that beyond the age of 45, we lose about 1% of muscle mass per year, meaning that by age 65, we may have lost about 20% of our muscle mass if not exercising. And losing muscle mass decreases stability and increases the chances of falls, resulting in fractures, especially around the hips.

Astoundingly, we have over 650 muscles in our bodies. Because there are so many and because they give our bodies incredible support, it is vital that we continuously strengthen our muscles through exercise. Strength and conditioning training is the perfect way to get our muscles in shape and keep them working correctly.

Our muscles are grouped into three basic categories; skeletal, smooth, and cardiac muscles.

Skeletal muscles

They are so named because most skeletal muscles move the skeleton's bones. However, a few skeletal muscles are synergists, meaning they don't directly impact the bones but assist other muscles. Through alternating contraction and relaxation or sustained contraction, muscles play a vital function in the body. For example, they stabilize our bodies, produce heat (to normalize body temperature), facilitate the movement of nutrients in the body, and aid blood flows back to the heart.

Skeletal muscles are the most common muscles in our bodies, taking on a wide range of functions, as mentioned above. If we don't take care of these, we are well on the road toward muscle injuries and diseases. In addition, age-related degeneration, strains, falls, and fractures are common problems related to weakened skeletal muscles.

Smooth muscles

These muscles are called "smooth" because they don't have striations (alternating dark and light bands) when viewed under a microscope, unlike skeletal and cardiac muscles. They are found in blood vessels, urinary bladder, reproductive tracts, and the gut. Their action is involuntary, and some, like the gut, have auto-rhythmicity.

Examples of typical smooth muscles are our intestines and the inner walls of our blood vessels. While it's impossible to actively and directly train smooth muscles, we can improve their capacity through exercise - albeit indirectly. For example, training the cardiovascular system improves blood and nutrient supply to the smooth muscles, boosting their health.

Cardiac muscles

These are muscles of the heart. When they contract, they pump blood from the heart to the rest of the body. The heart's alternating contraction and relaxation functions are not controlled consciously. Instead, the heart has a pacemaker that initiates contractions producing the beats. These contractions are in-built rhythms called auto-rhythmicity.

Some hormones can adjust the pace at which the heart beats. For example, the heart slows down when the body releases the acetylcholine hormone. Conversely, when the adrenaline hormone is released, the heart beats fast.

"Sitting disease" is the new name for our chronic lack of inactivity. Studies show that weakened cardiac muscles resulting from too much sitting increases our risk of heart disease, high blood pressure, and diabetes.

As you can see, muscle health dramatically contributes to our overall health. Healthy muscles offload the joints, slowing the progression of osteoarthritis. They also prevent the twisting movement of the joints, which may lead to fractures and tears of ligaments. For example, we have three muscles at the back of the thigh (hamstrings), and they all cross the knee joint, attaching to the leg bones (tibia and fibula).

One tendon (the biceps femoris tendon) attaches to the fibula. The semitendinosus tendon grabs the side of the tibia. And the semimembranosus tendon attaches to the back of the tibia. If there is muscle weakness of the three muscles in different proportions, whichever force is more powerful will cause a twisting action. And our joints don't enjoy twisting at all!

Studies show that having healthy muscles increases our lifespan. Healthy chest muscles enable us to breathe correctly, delivering adequate oxygen supply to body tissues and preventing hypostatic pneumonia (a type of pneumonia common in weak or bedridden elderly patients). Conversely, muscle loss produces delayed wound healing, lower resting metabolic rate, physical impairment, lower quality of life, increased healthcare costs, and mortality.

So how does strength and conditioning training help our muscles get stronger?

The purpose of strength and conditioning exercises is to improve the body's metabolic processes, making our bodies more robust and efficient. According to research, short bouts of frequent strength training can boost muscle growth.

When we use our muscles in a manner that is different from how we use them daily, our bodies naturally respond to adapt by getting stronger. For example, lifting weights builds strength because our muscles are required to work harder than usual; doing pushups forces your arms, shoulders, and chest to work harder at keeping you up than they would be otherwise; and a simple jog around the block can help strengthen your heart.

And while we are still on muscles, S&C training has been proven to increase lean muscle, reducing inflammation (Chapter 5 discusses lean muscles in detail). An analysis of this theory shows that smaller fat cells found in leaner individuals create healthier body functions. On the contrary, enlarged fat cells in less lean people lead to chronic illnesses, pains, aches, and inflammations.

It's more difficult for fat to be broken down and converted to energy with less lean muscle.

The fewer lean muscles we have, the less fat we can break down for energy. Less lean muscle will also reduce metabolic processes that lead to inflammation, resulting in less fatigue. As a result, you can train harder, increase your fitness levels, and improve your health and well-being.

2. Helps Core/Balance, Mobility, Posture, Injury Prevention

What are core muscles?

These muscles support the pelvis, stomach, buttocks, back, and hips. The central core muscles are:

- Rectus abdominis muscles (the six-packs)
- Multifidus (deep lower back muscle)
- Transverse abdominal (lower abs)
- Erector spinae (a muscle that runs along the spine)
- Diaphragm (dome-shaped muscle below the ribcage)
- Inner and outer obliques (muscles that help us rotate side to side)
- Pelvic floor muscles (they form the base of the pelvis and control incontinence)

So, now that you know core muscles aren't just the celebrated "six-pack" ab muscles around your stomach, you can understand how important they are. When all these muscles around our backs, sides, and torsos, particularly those wrapped around the spine, are strengthened, they "hold us up" and keep us upright. Moreover, the improved posture that follows a reinforced core can reduce irksome lower backache, hamstring strains, groin pulls, and neck pain. According to studies, a strong core is vital to developing good posture and reduces our risk of injury by 30%.

The bottom line is that stronger core muscles improve balance and mobility. When doing your exercises from a solid base, it's easier to hold yourself upright even when the ground is unsteady or recover quickly after a misstep. When the core muscles around the midsection are strong, they automatically create an equilibrium in our bodies. We can stand a little taller, hold steady for longer, lift more, and maintain a solid form as we move. When the muscles around our mid-section are more powerful, there is less rocking, movement, and energy dissipated, allowing for the smooth and uniform working of the pelvis, lower back, and hips.

And let's not forget that most vital organs are right below the abdominal wall. When the muscles around this area are strong, they act as a shield against anything external. So the more robust our core muscles are, the more protective they are of the internal organs.

3. Increases Energy and Endurance

Strength and conditioning training can also help increase energy levels. It improves the heart, lungs, and muscles and allows us to maintain strength and athleticism as we grow older. In addition, the exercises themselves can significantly affect the cardiovascular system.

When we exercise, our bodies produce extra mitochondria inside our muscle cells. Mitochondria are organelles in body cells that produce energy from glucose in our meals. Having more of these organelles increases the energy available in our bodies.

Exercising also improves our bodies' oxygen circulation. This boost in oxygen helps the mitochondria produce more energy, helps our bodies work better and uses energy more efficiently. Additionally, our bodies benefit from increased hormone levels caused by exercise, which makes us feel much more invigorated. These hormones are known as endorphins or feel good hormones. They interact with our brain receptors in complex ways, reducing pain awareness, even during strenuous exercises. In addition, these feel-good hormones trigger positive feelings, which improve our mood, self-confidence, and sleep, all while reducing stress, anxiety, and the risk of depression.

4. Boosts Metabolism, Burns Fat, and Calories

Strength and conditioning workouts help us lose weight, gain muscle and get stronger. In addition, a disciplined routine can help us burn more calories throughout the day, which boosts our metabolism and helps melt extra fat.

Because muscle burns more calories than fat, we will burn more calories the more muscles we have. We need some fat for energy, but our body shouldn't have too much as this can lead to inflammation and disease. Via consistent S&C training, unhealthy fat will convert to muscle, which gives us better overall body control.

5. Makes Bones Stronger

According to Wolff's law, bones respond to the amount of stress placed on them. Therefore, regular S&C training causes an increase in bone density because it increases the pressure on our skeletal system. When there is increased stress on the bones, they respond by making new connective tissue to reinforce them.

Strength training increases the density of bones by causing microscopic damage to them. This statement might sound counterintuitive, but this action stimulates the body to lay down new bone. Strength training is, therefore, a great way to prevent osteoporosis, reduce the risk of falls, and improve the overall quality of life.

6. Injury, Pain, and Disease Recovery

Whether we have a severe or minor injury, a quick recovery is our first objective. Recovery from injury is critical for muscle healing and strength building. A severe injury, especially one that limits mobility, can negatively impact our lives.

We may not achieve our best fitness objectives when injured, but resistance workouts can help us to heal faster. The most common injuries that affect the musculoskeletal system are dislocations, strains, sprains, fractures, and spasms.

S&C training is essential in injury rehabilitation programs as the process promotes tissue healing by stimulating blood circulation. Improved blood circulation ensures enough oxygen and nutrients are transported to all body tissues. In this way, strength training promotes healing, so you can quickly return to the activities you love doing sooner. Most importantly, regular strength training helps prevent injuries by improving our range of motion and balance to stay steady on our feet, even at higher speeds and on unstable surfaces.

By strengthening the muscles, ligaments, tendons, and bones, S&C training helps hold the body upright and in proper alignment. Under impact or during movement, stronger ligaments, muscles, and tendons protect the body and joints from fractures. In addition, S&C training improves bone strength by placing overloads on them recurrently.

Moreover, S&C training improves the flexibility of the ligaments so they can act as efficient shock absorbers where dynamic movements are involved.

S&C training is beneficial for joints. Remember, strength training builds muscles that support the joints. So building muscle is a critical part of joint pain management, and most physicians will recommend it, whether you have osteoarthritis, psoriatic arthritis, inflammation, or any autoimmune disorder.

Think of a sapling fruit tree and imagine your joint as one. Saplings are weak and delicate. To grow straight and strong, you must tie strings around them; without the lines, they don't stand a chance. The same thing applies to joints; they need the support of muscles and ligaments. With the strong strings, the sapling plant thrives and bears enough fruit. Still, the same applies to joints. Without the support of strong muscles, they will take a pounding sooner or later.

As you engage and strengthen the muscles around the joints through S&C conditioning, they "master the art" of absorbing extra force, taking the pressure off the worn-out joints. This shift can significantly reduce joint stiffness and provide relief from pain.

Rheumatology, a scientific publication, recently highlighted the importance of strong muscles for joint function. According to the report, strong muscles ease pain caused by osteoarthritis while improving their general function. Another Finnish report backed up these findings and proved that 59% of early rheumatoid arthritis patients who did S&C training at least twice a week for 24 months saw a positive shift in morning stiffness, joint pain, and inflammation compared to those who didn't.

7. Enhances Mental Health

S&C training affects mental health in several ways. First, it helps reduce stress and anxiety. Improving our physical state will help increase our confidence, a key component in maintaining a positive mood. It also releases endorphins, the chemical responsible for giving us a sense of well-being after finishing an exercise routine or exercising in general. Strength training is proven to boost our moods by stimulating the brain through movement.

By strengthening our physical health through an exercise routine, we begin to see benefits in other areas of life. For example, as we lose weight and become stronger physically, we may notice that we also feel happier and have less stress because we love the results in the mirror.

8. Increases Cognitive Brain Function

Strength and conditioning play an essential role in cognitive function. Cognitive function is the ability to comprehend and learn new information, store it in long-term memory and retrieve it when needed. Strength training improves mental function by improving brain health, which leads to improved neuroplasticity, which can lead to improved thinking skills and problem-solving ability.

The relationship between strength and conditioning and cognitive function is vital. For example, research from the National Institute of Health found that fitness helps memory; this study analyzed the effects of fitness on middle-aged participants' ability to remember words and names. The results showed a direct correlation between physical fitness and cognitive performance, suggesting that maintaining a healthy lifestyle will reduce our risk of dementia in later life.

So, S&C training positively affects brain function. Our bodies release hormones (pregnenolone, testosterone, and estrogen) that improve memory when we exercise. Additionally, cardiovascular exercise boosts blood flow to the brain, which provides oxygen-rich nutrients to the neurons in our brain. We could prevent, slow down or reverse cognitive decline with strength and cardiovascular training.

9. Improves Sleep

Recent research shows that strength and conditioning training is a great way to improve our mental and physical health. It greatly benefits our sleep because if we feel more energized and less stressed, we're more likely to get a good night's rest. In addition, the healthier we are physically and cognitively, the easier it becomes to sleep more deeply and for more extended periods.

Strength and conditioning is one of the most fruitful ways to improve sleep quality and ease fatigue. A new study at the University of Maryland and Old Dominion University found that older adults who did high-intensity strength training for four months significantly improved their sleep quality than those who did low-intensity weight lifting or cardiovascular exercise.

Resistance training improves sleep because building muscles takes energy and that, in turn, requires rest at night. Moreover, building muscle uses up testosterone, which can prolong sleep. Also, serotonin (a neurotransmitter) is released in the brain after physical activity and aids in healthy sleep.

10. More Aging Fighting Benefits: Blood Pressure, Digestion, Hormone Levels, Heart Health (via Cardio Exercises), Controls Inflammation, Improves Digestion, Improves Skin, Blood Sugar

Many studies have proven the positive results of S&C on reducing blood pressure. It does this by strengthening the muscles that surround our arteries. In some cases, the increase in muscle strength contributes to reducing stress hormones, such as adrenaline and cortisol, which are known to increase blood pressure.

Strength and conditioning training has been demonstrated to improve digestion, especially for people with digestive issues or gastric pain. In addition, simple stretching before and after meals helps to keep our bodies limber, resulting in less physical stress on the digestive organs that can cause stomach cramps and pain.

Regular strength training also tends to make us feel fuller, so we end up eating less food. This feeling can help prevent overindulging in unhealthy foods and sweets, which may cause bloating, cramps, and other digestive problems. It also increases the odds that our bodies will absorb more nutrients from food, which helps keep our intestines healthy.

According to studies, evidence is clear that strength and conditioning training has a positive effect on hormone levels:

- **Dopamine** - resistance exercises increase the dopamine hormone levels, reducing stress and depression.
- **Testosterone** - this hormone is linked to physical strength, heart health, metabolism, and bone and muscle mass. Testosterone levels decline as we age, but strength training increases these levels, helping us battle aging.
- **Estrogen** - estrogen levels drop at the onset of menopause. Strength training increases estrogen levels and alleviates postmenopausal symptoms.
- **Serotonin** - is a hormone and a neurotransmitter that tells your brain how to respond to different stimuli. Conditioning and strength training increases serotonin levels, stabilizing your mood.

Studies show that S&C helps lower blood sugar by forcing our bodies into an anabolic mode. This process means that more glucose gets stored as glycogen in your muscles instead of being stored as fat, subsequently reducing the risk of diabetes by improving blood sugar control and fat gain through weight loss.

Moreover, strength training also improves insulin sensitivity allowing for better carbohydrate metabolism and utilization. Strength training builds muscle, and research has shown that the more muscle tissue you have in your body, the better your body can handle carbohydrates. It also reduces cardiovascular risk by lowering blood pressure directly related to Type 2 Diabetes.

Strength and conditioning training reduces inflammation by promoting a natural anti-inflammatory status in the body. It fights inflammation by changing how the brain interprets pain signals from tissues. Strength training also battles inflammation by increasing muscle and tissue blood flow. The increased blood flow brings more nutrients, oxygen, and white blood cells to areas of the body experiencing pain or discomfort. Also, exercise helps break down adhesions, scar tissue, fibrin, and other harmful by-products of inflammation.

Amazingly, strength training is also excellent for your skin. It can keep the skin healthy and youthful. Recent studies on the benefits of strength training show that exercises improve our skin's elasticity and thickness. When stretched, an elastic skin has more capacity to return to its original state. In addition, S&C training improves blood circulation, which increases the delivery of oxygen and nutrients to skin cells.

When you complete a workout, you feel good. Our bodies produce endorphins during exercise. Endorphins are feel-good hormones. When we feel good, our stress levels reduce. Stress is a normal part of life, but chronic stress is bad for the skin. Chronic stress has connected to many skin problems, including acne, psoriasis, and symptoms of atopic dermatitis. Looking at it this way, we would all agree that exercise is good for our skin.

A study by the National Sleep Foundation reports that people who exercise sleep better. Getting enough sleep every night is good for your skin and helps reduce overall stress levels, which is also good for the skin. Exercise helps the skin both directly and indirectly, as highlighted here.

Over the last few decades, experts have spent more time studying the benefits of S&C training, and their findings have been astonishing. For example, analysis of data from the National Health Interview Survey of adults 65 years and older, those who took on strength and condition training at least twice a week had up to 46% reduced odds of death compared to their peers who didn't do any S&C exercises.

They lowered their risk of cardiac arrest by up to 41% and the odds of dying a cancer-related death by 19%. In addition, in the eye-opening results of the study, it was reported that there were direct links between S&C training to other healthier habits. For example, the same adults who did strength and conditioning exercises twice a week were more likely to be well-educated, be within a healthy weight range, didn't consume alcohol or smoke cigarettes, and are actively involved in aerobic exercises.

When the researchers adjusted variables such as demographics, health conditions, and behaviors, the results favored seniors actively involved in S&C training. When they changed physical activity levels, seniors who did S&C training still had lower mortality rates than those who only did physical activities like aerobics.

This study in and of itself should prove that the benefits of strength and condition training aren't just limited to physical function or muscle and bone strength. Instead, the benefits could be the difference between life and death.

So, here we have more than ten excellent strength and conditioning training benefits! Hopefully, you gravitated toward some of these and can start recognizing the importance of applying S&C to your daily routine. Starting something new that requires effort is usually not easy. But nothing worthwhile usually is. In this next chapter, we'll talk about how to apply this information and create an excellent health and fitness lifestyle.

Chapter 3
The Approach: Mindset and Motivation

"There is a fountain of youth: it is your mind, your talents, the creativity you bring to your life and the lives of people you love. When you learn to tap this source, you will truly have defeated age."

- Sophia Loren

STARTING THE JOURNEY

While this book provides a practical template of strength and conditioning exercises and workouts, I must acknowledge that starting something new like this can often be a real struggle. Especially something physical. But, we can mitigate the battle immensely by ensuring we start with a proper mindset and motivation.

For the sake of the next point, let's consider the Ironman triathletes when they first decided to compete at an elite level. They didn't just snap their fingers and were instantly able to swim, run and bike a grueling 140.6 miles. Instead, they first decided that being an elite-level athlete was something they wanted, still knowing that it could be an excruciating journey. Ironman training is extremely tough, and I guarantee that each athlete pursuing that level of training counts the cost. Yet their initial decision to pursue it had to start from somewhere. It had to have a genesis that would propel them into laying a successful framework to complete their mission.

All elite athletes who attempt Ironman competitions have two things in common before they start training. The first is that they believe they can do it. One of the most challenging parts of any training is the beginning. And these elite triathletes all start with "belief." And the second thing they have in common is motivation. Motivation to see the necessary training and competitions through to completion. So having a belief and motivation is where the process begins and starts the hardwiring process in our minds.

It's about programming our brains to tell our bodies that we're going to do something different, something challenging, and something potentially physically demanding and internalizing it. Now please understand that at-home workouts with this book won't be even remotely as grueling as training for an Ironman triathlon. This book and these workouts are simply a starter's guide to strength and conditioning training. However, the motivation principles to accomplish our missions are the same…identical.

FINDING MOTIVATION, THE "WHYS"

As you might imagine, the exercise journey is more than just picking up a weight willy-nilly and going through the motions of a workout regiment. Just like the triathlete, it first starts with our belief that we can do it. This belief fuels our motivation to help us begin a new system, allows us to make gains, and helps us stay consistent. Our motivation drives us not to give up after a few weeks, a few days, or even a few hours.

Multiple studies have proven that new experiences are good for our brains. The experiences reshape and rejuvenate our thinking. But why do we often stop something we've wholeheartedly told ourselves we really wanted? It's because our excuses outweigh our desires, which means we haven't established reasons sticky enough to keep us going. The good news is that there is *always* something inside ourselves that can provide this motivation to help us stay the course. We just have to find "it."

For this reason, we must establish our mindset before or when we begin training. We all know that along the way, life will always (not can, will) throw us some curveballs, delivering many temptations that can steer us away from our prize…if we let them. In these moments, we need to have a hearty mindset to recall and lean on why we're doing what we've initially determined to do. Merriam-Webster's Dictionary defines mindset as 1) a mental attitude or inclination, 2) a fixed state of mind. Therefore, ensuring our "mind is set" on our objectives before we begin is paramount.

I'm going to go out on a limb here and say that by picking up this book, we've already established that our overarching, most general "why" is to combat aging, right? If we boil it all down to the beginning, your mindset is already on the right path if you're reading this book. You have planted the seed. But let's take it a step further and quickly revisit the additional "whys" we outlined in Chapter 1 and the many "benefits" for strength and conditioning outlined in Chapter 2. These benefits will offer us added direction to finding our personal "whys." Here they are again, the 10+ benefits of strength and conditioning training:

- Strengthens and builds lean muscles
- It helps balance, mobility, posture, and injury prevention
- Increases energy and endurance
- Boosts metabolism, burns fat and calories
- Makes bones stronger
- Helps with injury, pain, and disease recovery
- Enhances our mental health

- Increases cognitive brain function
- Improves sleep
- Aids blood pressure, digestion, hormones, inflammation, skin, etc.

What a list of benefits, right?! Can you see why we needed to review all of these? This information provides an excellent foundation for motivation, which is where we need to go next.

Now it's time to dig deeper and discover our personal "whys." We now need to anchor our mindset, which will drive our hard work, so we won't stop until we lose those extra pounds, break that sweat, push our limits and get in shape.

If we don't do this, we'll quickly resort to an "I'll *do it tomorrow*" when we feel lethargic, or the weather outside is unpleasant. All of us have experienced this. Everyone who has ever started something new faces the same issue every time they start. Soon "tomorrow" turns into days, then weeks, which can quickly snowball into months. An essential tactic that has proven to circumvent this "snowball effect" is never to forget the reason "why" you started.

The Story of Mario Lemieux

Growing up in Wisconsin, I knew a little bit about hockey. Although, I honestly didn't know much as I spent most of my winters training and competing in the sport of wrestling. However, I did know about NHL great Mario Lemieux (phonetically pronounced leh-MYOO), one of the best and most storied hockey players of all time.

What made Mario so great (fans called him Super Mario) is still somewhat of a secret, as with many other great athletes. Oddly enough, when asked, they often struggle to define what makes them great. However, this story isn't about what made Mario great (or super). Instead, it's about his "why."

In 1997, 31-year-old Mario Lemieux retired from hockey with incredible accolades. Born and raised in Quebec, he was the first pick in the first round of the 1984 draft by the Pittsburgh Penguins. He became rookie of the year in his first season, and in the first six seasons, he scored more than 100 points. Only a few years later, he was named Most Valuable Player (MVP) of the National Hockey League (NHL). Devastatingly, Mario missed 54 games in the 1991 season for back surgery that he had in the off-season to fix a herniated disc. However, he remarkably returned to help the team win a Stanley Cup Championship and earn playoff MVP honors. Then in the next season, he led the Penguins to another Stanley Cup Championship, and Lemieux won another MVP.

In 1993 Mario was diagnosed with Hodgkin's disease halfway through the season. He missed 20 games for radiation treatment yet still won the league's top scorer and MVP honors that year. The following season he sat out 22 games to recover from his cancer treatment and ongoing back issues, including surgery to try and fix a herniated muscle. The two-time champion's future started looking bleak. Amazingly, Lemieux managed to muster a recovery, join the 1995-6 season, and still lead the league in scoring, winning a third MVP award. But wait, there's more.

In 1997 Lemieux went on to win his sixth scoring title while starting to wrestle again with health issues. Finally, it seemed that his cancer treatment and its consequent effects on how he wanted to perform on the ice forced him to retire at 31. That year, the Hockey Hall of Fame expeditiously inducted Lemieux due to all the accomplishments packed into his short career. This is where the story gets good.

A year after his induction into the Hall of Fame, the Pittsburgh Penguins started feeling the effects of Mario's departure. Oddly enough, they had already been in a financial pickle and continued to slide, declaring bankruptcy in 1998. Lamenting a possible purchase and move of the Pittsburgh franchise, Mario decided to convert much of his unpaid salary from the Penguins into equity. He then found some investors to help him buy the team. Additionally, Mario decided to come out of retirement for the 2001 season and became the first-ever player-owner in NHL history! That season he went on to take The Penguins to the playoffs, was named to the NHL All-Star team, and heroically saved the future of the Penguin's franchise.

There were many achievements Mario Lemieux garnered in his professional hockey career, from his five Stanley Cup Championships (two as a player and three as an owner) to multiple MVPs, scoring titles, and All-Star teams. But again, let's not focus here on what he won specifically and what made him great, but on his "why." Why do you think Mario returned to become the first-ever player-owner after all his physical hardships? What drove him to not rest on his laurels and retire after the accomplishments (and millions of dollars earned) for a comfortable life?

Mario Lemieux's "why" was to help save the Penguin franchise and thousands of Pittsburgh fans' hearts in the process. The team that was near and dear to him, who picked him first in the draft, and where he stayed his entire hockey career, was financially collapsing. Had he not stepped in, the Penguins could have easily landed in another city other than Pittsburgh. His affection for his team and his fans was his "why" and is what motivated him to mount one of the most storied comebacks in modern sports history.

While you and I will never manage an NHL comeback as Lemieux did, we still need to find out our "why" if we are ever going to do something incredibly challenging. Making a lifestyle change like starting a new exercise program will not be easy. But discovering our "why," like Mario Lemieux did, will provide a core reason to keep us driving forward and coming back.

So, what is YOUR motivation? What is your "why." Is it weight, better skin, disease prevention, wanting to be around for our grandkids, trying to win the heart of a fair maiden, etc.? Is it a combination of things? Whatever "it" is, I would strongly encourage you to find it, write it down and internalize it daily. I'll show you exactly how to start doing this later in the chapter.

MINDSET FOR MOTIVATION

Mindset - Fixed vs. Growth

As we explore motivation here, I want to be sure to acknowledge two different types of thinking to ensure we're all fully equipped. We've already established that after we decide to take the plunge into something challenging, we must first establish the foundation of a "proper mindset" (especially for older adults who, let's not kid ourselves, tend to be set in their ways). But what is a "proper mindset"? What determines a kind of mindset that's effective? To answer that, we first answer a fundamental question, "are we fixed in our ways (in our minds), or do we want to grow"?

According to Carol Dweck, a behavioral psychologist from Stanford, what you believe in significantly impacts your failure or success rate. And it's not our genetics or the environment that limits our learning potential. A few years of commitment, training, and toil could set us for a brighter future, but only if we can cultivate a belief that we can do it, which is a positive mindset, a "growth mindset."

Someone with a growth mindset tends to believe in their abilities, talents, capabilities, and the possibility of growth through passion, perseverance, and persistence. Of course, this isn't about thinking that we can become the next Martin Luther King Jr, Mozart, or Albert Einstein; better if we can. Still, it's about entertaining the thought that anyone can become better if they are genuinely committed and work toward it.

A fixed mindset assumes intelligence, character, and ability are predetermined and can never be changed. It's even worse when a fixed mindset conditions someone to think that effort isn't required and success relies only on talent and intelligence. Unchecked, the fixed mindset can impact and control all areas of our lives.

A growth mindset embraces new challenges while a fixed mindset shies away from them. A growth mindset doesn't view failure as an indication of intelligence but as a revitalizing springboard that helps it stretch its abilities.

So do you think you can change? If so, you must fight that inner voice that harkens back to a fixed mindset and replace it with visualizations of success and positive self-talk for growth. We can condition our minds just like our bodies. And a growth mindset is where we start; without it, no workout program will work, no matter how effective it is on paper.

The Mindset of Elon Musk

Many people today know who Elon Musk is, a multi-billionaire with a long list of incredible business successes. But he wasn't always this person. Some know he's from South Africa, born in 1971, and lived in Canada for a few years before moving to the United States.

Most don't know that Elon struggled early in his life, being bullied and was incredibly lonely as a child. In a recent article, his mother, Maye Musk, is quoted as saying, "Elon was the youngest and smallest guy in his school" and that he was picked on constantly. And in early adulthood, he often bounced from one odd job to the next before going to college in 1992.

Fast forward to 2002. Elon sold his technology company Paypal to eBay for $1.5 billion. That year he also started SpaceX, a space exploration company that works jointly with NASA. And then, in 2003, Musk created Tesla, arguably one of the most innovative automobile manufacturing companies in history.

Now, Musk has some incredible intelligence to advance his success as fast as he did. He attended the University of Pennsylvania and earned physics and economics degrees, so he was no dummy. But one of the main differences between Musk and average individuals is that his mindset became entirely focused on making his giant ideas happen.

Elon Musk once said,

"If you want to grow a giant redwood, you need to make sure the seeds are ok, nurture the sapling, and work out what might potentially stop it from growing all the way along. Anything that breaks it at any point stops that growth."

Can the average person think the same way? Yes, why not? However, we must cultivate the correct "growth" mindset. We must train our thoughts as we set a target for ourselves, making sure our "seeds" are ok, nurturing our "saplings," and "work out" what might stop our growth. Every successful person has some version of this mindset. They cherish their tree and make it a priority to protect its growth.

MOTIVATION PRINCIPLES

According to a 1991 study by researchers John Arnold, Ivan Robertson, and Cary Cooper, motivation has three core components. These are; direction, intensity, and persistence. Direction is where you've chosen to go, whether to exercise (or watch TV). Intensity is the level at which you choose to participate in that direction, and persistence is the ability to stick with your direction and intensity.

An article by Jim Taylor, Ph.D. called the Power of Prime, is about how vitally clear motivation is for athletes to succeed. In the article, he made the results of the study previously mentioned by Arnold, Robertson, and Cooper a bit easier to remember. He lists the three components as the three D's; Direction, Decision, and Dedication.

So why is it important to know about these three components? Well, at the very least, it reveals three distinct links in our thought process chain where our desire to combat aging could go wrong. But, at the very best, it lets us know that if these three components work in harmony, we can almost guarantee that our endeavors will succeed.

While these three components are essential to understand, they only really benefit us if we develop some specific strategies to keep them in harmony. So let's move on to explore some of these to help keep our Direction, Decision, and Dedication intact.

Find your "Whys":

Write down the specific reasons why you want to do this. As iterated earlier, without a compelling "why," we'll find a reason to procrastinate or quit altogether. Remember, you have what it takes to do this. A powerful "why" is essential because:

- It pushes us to increase our effort and boost productivity.
- It inspires people around us to do more.
- It fuels our habits.
- It gives us a reason to work towards our dreams and goals.

- It helps us adopt a positive mindset as we work toward those goals.
- It opens our minds to the possibilities.

It's almost impossible to achieve success without a clear "why."

Make Goals

Write down short- and long-term goals, and dream or visualize where you want to be. Write down the specifics of what you want to achieve and within what timeframe. It could be as easy as losing 1 pound in a week or a month, walking 2 miles daily, etc.

Set goals that increase your odds of success and achievement. They should focus on productivity, efficiency, and how much time you have. As you write down your goals, ensure all your ideas are clarified, and your efforts are focused on the task.

You've probably heard this acronym before, but I must emphasize that our goals should be Specific, Measurable, Attainable, Real, and Time-bound (SMART).

Specific: When it comes to the goal's specifics, you must ask yourself the 5 Ws questions: what, why, when, which, and where.

Measurable: How many goals will you set, and how are you tracking your accomplishments?

Attainable: Are the goals realistic and realizable?

Real: Do you think the goal is worth pursuing? If yes, is now the right time to pursue it in that specific environment? Are you well-prepared to do whatever it takes?

Time-Bound: When it comes to time-bound, we must ask ourselves, how much can I achieve today, in a week, month, or six months?

Goals give us clarity and the motivation we need to go after what we want. And when you learn how to make them and use them well as one of your tools, you can transfer your goal-making system to anything else you want to accomplish.

Celebrate Victories

Small victories (and victories of any size, for that matter) must be celebrated. You're on a journey. Have fun while you're on it, and have fun when you've reached your destinations! But then it's done, and you're on to the next one!

It's important to celebrate small wins; if we don't, we may lose the motivation and drive to go on. Success works this way:

Taking action -> Achievement -> Happiness -> Celebration -> Taking more action -> More achievement

Taking action -> Achievement -> Happiness -> No celebration -> Less motivation -> Less action -> Less results -> Less achievement.

You may not achieve everything you want the way you want and whenever you want, but it's essential to celebrate when you do.

Here are some ideas to celebrate your achievements:

- Buy yourself something- a gift?
- Write down your achievement.
- Acknowledge your achievement
- Share your joy with others.
- You can make it a little event if you are in a position to
- Practice gratitude
- Take a break and do something you love and enjoy
- You can create a recognition award to celebrate your victory

Form Good Habits

Form habits to help you stay on track and persistent.

Habits are powerful: they can determine success or failure. So the first step toward improving our productivity and making our lives easier is to develop good habits. So how do we do that?

Understanding how our habits shape our behaviors is essential.

1. So, let's say you've identified a goal. The goal should spur you into daily action. It can be either short-term or long-term.
2. Find a routine that works for you. For example, if you plan on jogging or going for a run, you can choose a morning or evening routine.
3. Create a trigger that reminds you of what needs to be done. An alarm clock or phone alarm is an effective trigger. Do this long enough, and you'll create a habit.

Good habits are created over time, so you must be strong-willed and stay the course until you achieve your objective.

Welcome Correction

Find a coach/accountability partner and get feedback on your progress. There are HUGE benefits to this. According to *Better Than Before*, author Gretchen Rubin says, "External accountability works best." Rubin highlights the importance of accountability in making and breaking habits in his book. For example, you are more likely to achieve an S&C goal (or any other goal) if you work with a trainer or a fitness partner.

If you'd rather be your own accountability "police," you can use an app that tracks progress and gives reminders. You can also create an accountability journal or calendar and make daily entries. According to one weight loss study by North Carolina State University, participants who had buddy support lost more weight along their waistline than those who didn't.

Only a few people can be accountable to themselves, but most need that external push to get things done. So please do what you must to achieve your goal: from choosing an accountability partner to changing bad habits and negative mindsets.

Believe in yourself

Many people indeed struggle with self-doubt and negativity. Still, we've also heard amazing stories of successful people who excelled because they believed in themselves, their talents, and abilities even when no one else did.

Most know Muhammad Ali as one of the greatest boxers of all time. Ali pretty much sums up the idea of believing in yourself in a simple quote, "*He who is not courageous enough to take risks will accomplish nothing in life.*" Ali said this not because he didn't have moments of self-doubt or failure but because his desire to win surpassed the risks and setbacks that resulted from his failures.

Many people are paralyzed to inaction by fear of failure and are obsessed with their need for perfectionism. I know because I often struggle with this myself. If you do too, then you understand that we have trouble coping with needing everything "just right" before moving forward. This action is often a guise for fear and can often prevent us from living life to the fullest by not taking risks. We fear making mistakes. Unfortunately, when we do this, we end up in the wrong mindset, stuck with indecision, tension, and being too cautious.

So please be mindful that we don't succeed because we've never failed; we succeed despite failures. We must strive to get over our need for perfection to eliminate self-doubt and fear of failure. You can do this. You have everything right inside of you to make this happen.

Be Realistic

According to recent studies, people with an optimistic and realistic outlook are happier, healthier, and more successful. A sensible approach is practical and better for your mental health. Many self-help books promote the message of realistic and positive thinking.

Normal Vincent Peale's bestselling book, The Power of Positive Thinking, claims: "*When you expect the best, you release a magnetic force in your mind which by a law of attraction tends to bring the best to you.*"

This approach isn't about having an unrealistically rosy viewpoint or overlooking today's hardships. Instead, it is about launching a self-fulfilling prophecy where you don't need anything more than self-belief to succeed. A winning mindset is a result of realistic optimism.

Unrealistic optimism other the other hand is defined as the inclination to overestimate the possibility that something good will happen while underrating the likelihood that something terrible might happen. It's a common human trait. Studies show that 80% of the general population display unrealistic optimism tendencies. This is why you and I must make simple, realistic goals and visions as we embark on this journey. This way, we are better placed to achieve success.

Make It a Priority

I don't think anyone could have defined priority better than the Merriam-Webster Dictionary. It defines priority as "*something given or meriting attention before competing alternatives.*" And making something a priority, particularly exercise, takes self-discipline. Of course, people have opinions of what it means to prioritize something, but I believe prioritization is not an intellectual but an emotional aspect of life.

Getting rid of something you'd prefer to keep and replacing it with something more meaningful takes commitment, focus, and discipline. Believing you need exercise, wanting to do it, saying "I must do it," and making it a priority in your life are two different things. Unfortunately, most people quit along the way, choosing to delay, duck and even avoid the tough choices altogether.

Sadly, avoiding the more challenging choices means no progress or growth, which results in stagnation. Priorities are powerful, giving you clarity while eliminating unnecessary distractions so you can put all your energy on things that truly matter.

Just Start

We've all been there, thinking about something endlessly, but never really getting to a point where we have mastered enough courage to get it done. You argue with your internal self, worry about meaningless things, get distracted, procrastinate, promise yourself that you'll start soon, and create other excuses to procrastinate again – then, without even noticing, you end up in this endless vicious cycle.

You draw the battle line; tell yourself that never again. Tell yourself that you are done with the excuses like, "I'll just start tomorrow," or "it's already too late in the day," or some other trivial reason. These excuses can kill us, and we need to get them out of our heads.

Suppose you set the alarm for 6:00 am and hit the snooze to 6:10 am. Now, you must start at 6:20 because you are already a few minutes in – after all, "there's no other choice." That d*mn snooze button!

The "I'll start next week," "I'll start on Monday," "I'll start tomorrow, or at 9:30" excuses are a well-known recipe for disaster. They are, without sugar-coating it, a recipe for failure. They never work.

Why would you wait for Monday or push it to a New Year's resolution if you want to do it? Stop waiting to be "ready," wallowing in the "I will start on Monday" mindset, but never really take action. Often the most challenging part is just starting. It gets easier with time once you agree both in mind and body to move forward. Take that step today!

Chapter 4

Baby Steps:

Setting Goals

"A good goal is like a strenuous exercise - it makes you stretch."

- Mary Kay Ash

We've all done it, especially as the new year rolls in. "This is my year!" "I will make things happen!" 'I must do better!" Then you grab a pen and a journal and scribble down everything you want to achieve by this month or the end of the year. You are newly inspired and 100% optimistic that everything will work out perfectly this time. It doesn't matter that you abandoned the same goals before February last year and the year before that, etc., etc., etc.

How does this feel?

Imagine waking up every other day and going to work just because you have to. Speaking to others aimlessly or because you've no other choice; exercising just because it's a box to check, having no goals, ambitions, or aspirations for yourself or anyone around you.

But what about living in the complete opposite of this reality?

While we often set goals and never follow through, it's still better to do it than not. I don't think Clement Stone's message couldn't have been more straightforward for us at this point in this book, "*Aim for the moon. If you miss, you'll land among the stars.*"

THE FRAMEWORK

There is so much more to goals than most of us realize:

1. They are a psychological tool. You may not know it, but goal-setting fuels motivation and gives you self-drive.
2. Goal-setting gives you purpose and adds meaning to your actions.
3. Goals give you a roadmap to reach a clear destination.

4. Goals provide us with perspective; the more efficient you do it, the more chances you have of achievement.
5. Goals influence our minds to change for the better and choose more innovative alternatives.

A goal-setter sees the bigger picture and the possibilities. Studies link people who set goals with higher self-discipline, autonomy, self-esteem, and self-confidence. The same studies have found a strong link between success and goal setting. Our brains love awards and praises.

This chapter will discuss the framework of goal setting, the benefits of setting goals, how to set them, and how you can implement those strategies in our S&C program. It will provide simple yet specific techniques to help start you on a path of healthy lifestyle changes.

Before we get into some practice steps for goal-setting, let's consider how some of the most influential people (both historical and current) have become successful.

Benjamin Franklin

Ben Franklin, an American pioneer in goal-setting, created a plan of 13 guidelines as a "life plan" when he was 20 years old. He charted the goals daily, and when the day was over, he put a dot by the ones at which he failed. While his goals weren't your average, run-of-the-mill resolutions, he charted these guidelines throughout his life. His goals were; temperance, silence, order, industry, cleanliness, tranquility, and humility.

In addition to this life plan, Franklin wrote down a rigorously detailed daily schedule. The model for it has transcended into what we know as the Franklin Planner, a paper-based time management system created by Richard Winwood and named after Franklin for his rigorous planning prowess.

Sara Blakely

Sara is an American entrepreneur and founder of Spanx, a brand that produces leggings, undergarments, and swimwear for women in more than 50 countries. She's a firm believer in writing down goals and visualizing them. After starting her business, Sara envisioned herself being on the Oprah show to promote her products, and in 2000, she did just that. Consequently, Oprah named her products one of her "favorite things." By 2012 she made the cover of Forbes magazine, which named her the youngest self-made female billionaire in the world. Today Sara is worth over $1.3 billion.

Richard Branson

Richard Branson is one of the wealthiest people on the planet and is best known for Virgin Records and Virgin Airlines. Branson faced many challenges in his early life, including dyslexia and ADHD, which made for some poor academic performance causing him to drop out of school. He also failed at many business ventures, including Virgin Publishing, Virgin Cars, and Virgin Cola, but is now worth about $4.5 billion and controls more than 400 companies within his Virgin Group conglomerate today. Branson attributes much of his success to his parents, failures, and his diligence with goal-setting. Branson created a 10-step goal-setting plan that brought him the success he now shares with other aspiring entrepreneurs.

Bruce Lee

In 1971 a relatively unknown man named Bruce Lee started having massive success as a martial artist movie character in China. Most don't know that a few years prior, Lee had written down on a piece of paper he titled "My Definite Chief Aim" that he'd be the highest-paid Oriental movie star in the US. These are the words he wrote:

"I, Bruce Lee, will be the first highest paid Oriental super star in the United States. In return, I will give the most exciting performances and render the best of quality in the capacity of an actor. Starting in 1970 I will achieve world fame and from then onward, till the end of 1980, I will have in my possession $10,000,000. I will live the way I please and achieve inner harmony and happiness." Bruce Lee, Jan. 1969

Bruce Lee died four years later but had already achieved his goal many times over. And his estate continues to make millions. Now, Lee is considered one of the biggest Hollywood martial arts legends.

From actors to business tycoons to 4-star generals, most will admit that one of the most critical ingredients (of their success) is goal-setting. But, as we all know, many things and distractions can derail our best intentions. That is why goal-setting is essentially an insurance policy for your success…and the only cost for the premium is your time to write them down and follow through with them.

The psychological definition of goal-setting

Goal-setting refers to the outlined plan of action intended to bring success. Goal-setting is the guiding light, the blueprint that sets us on the right path and ensures that we stay the course. In 1996, Edwin A. Locke, a pioneer in the goal-setting field, found a strong connection between people who set goals and those who excelled in their performance. According to his study, people who didn't set goals had a lower output rate than those who did.

Frank L. Small, Ph.D., has, for many years, studied the concept of goal setting in high-performing athletes and sportspeople. His findings have been astonishing; from them, he coined a three-letter phrase highlighting the essentials of goal setting. He called these essentials the A-B-Cs of goal-setting.

Small said that for a goal to be practical, it must also be:

A - Achievable

B - Believable

C - Committed.

As a psychological tool, goal-setting can improve productivity by involving George T. Doran's S-M-A-R-T approach. Doran proposed the idea of setting smart goals in his 1981 research paper. Over the years, the S-M-A-R-T goal concept has become one of the most popular concepts relating to goal-setting psychology.

We briefly discussed goal setting in chapter 3 when exploring how our mindset affects our success. Here we will break down what specific (SMART) goals look like, specifically regarding our strength and conditioning workouts.

But first, what would a SMART strength and conditioning workout goal look like?

It looks like setting a physical test or an S&C workout objective to be attained within a given time frame. The critical questions become:

What do you want to improve?

What would you like to achieve in the next few months?

How would you like to get this done?

Are you taking any steps to achieve this goal?

SMART goals are:

Specific

A specific goal should answer two primary questions…

- What do you want to accomplish?
- Why do you want to achieve it?

It can go even further and answer…

- Where and by when would you like to achieve the said goal?
- Will you need help from a coach, a trainer maybe?

Go for the bullseye, so you have a clear target at which to aim.

Here are examples of some specific goals:

- *"I want to gain more energy to climb the stairs without getting winded by the end of the month."*
- *'I want to gain at least 5 pounds of muscles by the end of the year."*
- *"I want to run a marathon with other seniors one year from now."*

Why?

- *"So I can hug my grandkids at the top of the stairs without having to catch my breath first."*
- *"So I can feel more nimble when I walk."*
- *"So I can improve my movements."*

Measurable

Will you measure your goal? How?

It will help if you can answer these questions...

- How many?
- How much?

Your measurable goals should be trackable to show how well you're progressing. It's the only way to monitor what you've achieved so far. We should gauge our measurable goals quantitatively or qualitatively.

Seeing how much progress you've made so far fuels and maintains your motivation. It can also show where improvement is needed and when it's time to set a new goal because you've achieved your last goal already.

A measurable goal looks something like this.

- "*I want to walk 50 more steps today than yesterday*" can be easily measured compared to "*I want to walk every day.*"
- "*I want to drink two more glasses of water each day*" is more measurable than "*I want to drink water every day.*"

Measurable goals help you monitor your progress once you have executed your plans.

Achievable

Is your goal reasonable? Is it individualized?

Understand that in exercise, particularly S&C training, no rule cuts across. Your goals should therefore consider this and be flexible in this regard. Don't set a goal that you know you might never accomplish. I know I said we should shoot for the moon, but if the goal is just "too much," you will struggle with motivation. You may have trouble maintaining your focus.

It will help if you start small and work your way up. You are the best barometer of what is realistic, so trust your instincts. For example, if you are just a beginner at exercising, you'll want to start slow, maybe 2-3 days a week, and add to it gradually.

Also, keep in mind that goals must be flexible. You can (and should) change them as often as you please. They should be fluid. And when you've achieved one, move on to the next one. It sounds simple, but being complacent after reaching a goal is common. So check that baby off and keep moving ahead!

Relevant/ Results-Based

Does this goal matter to you? Is it planned in a way that is easy to execute? Does the goal align with your long-term objectives?

We set goals not just to provide a plan but to provide something to execute. Therefore, if your goal doesn't match your longer-term objectives, it might not be necessary or relevant enough to include and measure.

You'll have a more challenging time trying to achieve a goal that doesn't align with or isn't meaningful to you. Besides, you don't want to overwork your body or overwhelm your metabolism by going after something that's not relevant. This isn't to say that some goals are unachievable, but it may take time, and it's essential to be aware of this.

Time-bound

What are the timelines for your goals?

Setting specific time increments will help "lock in" the other SMART components. Besides, time is an element that gives you more focus. Time-bound goals give you a time frame to achieve the task at hand.

For example:

- *"I will start drinking three glasses of water each morning in 5 days in the next week." Or,*
- *"I want to eliminate the nagging pain in my shoulder in 1 month by consistently stretching 5 or 10 minutes a day for the next month."*

Furthermore, a timeline gives you a basis for measurement, so you can observe if the achievement aligns with the deadline.

WHY ARE FITNESS GOALS IMPORTANT

- They improve our accountability.
- They motivate us to push past self-imposed barriers.
- They encourage us to look beyond temporary discomforts.
- Where possible, goals expand our vision and definition.
- We can work towards something meaningful.
- They boost our confidence.
- They give us a basis for self-evaluation by creating room for reflection and introspection.
- Achieving a goal gives us feelings of accomplishment and delight.

Did you know that goals shape the way we perceive others and ourselves? You are more likely to be an optimist if you are focused and goal-oriented than if you are not. You'll perceive failure as stepping stones, not weaknesses, as temporary setbacks than manifestations of your shortcomings.

Many studies have highlighted the benefits of goal setting, as mentioned throughout this chapter. The mind can be trained, and when we give it a clear vision to work towards and achieve, it rewires itself to obtain the best possible image, making the idea an essential part of our identity.

We feel good and have feelings of accomplishment when we achieve the goal, and if we don't, the brain, having been rewired, doesn't stop pushing us towards achievement until we finally do.

Researchers and psychologists encourage us to adopt SMART goal-setting techniques. Remember that we acquire skills over time, so it may take a while. The most important thing is to start. Don't be afraid to fail. It takes failure to be successful. NHL legend Wayne Gretzky sums it up pretty well, *"you miss one hundred percent of the shots you don't take"*

Irrational Goals - Don't Be Afraid

One disclaimer about the ABC or the SMART goals system is that these models sometimes need to be modified…similar to a mechanic who wants to modify an engine to go faster. As impressive as these goal frameworks are (especially for beginners), we need to ensure we don't box ourselves into something that's too rigid, especially as we exceed our expectations.

While SMART goals can be a solid basic structure to work within, we also need to be mindful that the "A" and the "R" letters in the acronym are still somewhat limiting…and on purpose. For example, the "A" for Achievable and the "R" for Realistic put some intentional constraints into the framework. George Doran originally designed these to prevent the goal-setter from becoming discouraged. And this is good because, more often than not, our small successes will help with our confidence, which in turn breeds more wins that get us to our goals. Additionally, it's sometimes a good idea not to bite off too much more than we can chew, especially when we're starting something new.

That said, if we bite off too much and fail, we learn much more than if we succeed. Don't we? Studies have proven that failure (not success) is often the better teacher. Failure is how we adapt and grow more quickly, as long as we are determined enough not to become discouraged. Many of the most successful people agree.

JK Rowling, the world's first billionaire author, said, "Failure gave me an inner security that I had never attained by passing examinations. Failure taught me things about myself that I could have learned no other way. I discovered I had a strong will and more discipline than I suspected." Thomas Edison said, "I have not failed. I have only found 10,000 ways that don't work." And Michael Jordan, the famous NBA superstar (who was demoted to the JV basketball team in high school), once said, "I've failed over and over again in my life, and that is why I succeed."

In other words, we shouldn't be afraid to set goals that might seem irrational. As humans, most of us don't grasp what we're truly capable of until we push ourselves to the limits. I'm not advocating this right out of the gate, but we need to ensure we're not limiting ourselves as we pick up momentum in reaching our goals. Let's consider this example for a moment to understand this point thoroughly.

Steve Jobs, co-founder, chairman, and CEO of Apple, was arguably one of the most innovative corporate leaders of our time. Not only was he a creative master, but he was also known for getting the most from his employees. While Jobs led by example, he also espoused a powerful philosophy that what they were working on made a massive difference in people's lives. Jobs was quoted as saying at Apple, "we attract a different type of person—a person who doesn't want to wait five or ten years to have someone take a giant risk on him or her. Someone who really wants to get in a little over his head and make a little dent in the universe." This statement essentially says, "we're going to bite off more than we can chew at our company."

There are many other examples of hugely successful CEOs who made irrational goals. Jeff Bezos, for instance, took Amazon from a company that sold books to the biggest online retailer in the world. Then there was Reed Hastings, who took Netflix from a DVD rental company to the biggest online streaming platform in the world.

Neither of these CEOs stayed entirely within a goal framework as it was their job to push beyond the limits of what was rational. They wanted to go further than what seemed realistic.

So while ABC or SMART systems are solid goal-setting frameworks that can work incredibly well, please keep in mind that to push yourself beyond what you think is possible, you shouldn't be afraid to consider goals that might seem unattainable. For example, if you are determined to be consistent and disciplined in your strength and conditioning workouts, you will probably be shocked by what you can accomplish.

Chapter 5
Two-Headed Monster:
Hydration & Nutrition

"Exercise is king. Nutrition is queen. Put them together and you've got a kingdom."

- Fitness and nutrition guru,
Jack LaLanne

Our bodies are like fine-tuned machines, working 24 hours a day, every day. The nutrients from our foods provide the fuel that keeps our bodies in motion and stabilizes us when we rest. So every day, we must eat nutritious foods containing proteins, vitamins, carbohydrates, minerals, and fats. And let's not forget water; it's a vital element of human nutrition.

You already know that as we age, our bodies change, and so do our nutritional needs. We may find that we now need more proteins, fewer fats, more vitamins, and mineral-rich foods. What we need to stay healthy in our senior years may be completely different from what we needed in our youth.

The National Resource Center on Nutrition, Physical Activity, and Aging reported that at least 25% of American seniors struggle with nutrition. Sadly, malnutrition leaves us vulnerable to muscle atrophy, reduced cognitive functions, and even disease. It can also leave us with weaker bones and increase the risk of being underweight or overweight.

You can already guess what I am driving at – we need more than just workouts to increase strength and build muscle tissue. Our bodies require nutrition to experience any change in their composition, like shedding off extra fat and replacing it with stronger muscles.

We might be extremely eager to get into the gym to become stronger, leaner, and more agile – that's great. However, we must focus on our nutrition as much as we do our S&C. We need to know what micro and macronutrients are, our calorie intake, what foods we should eat, and what foods we must avoid. And, of course, why hydration is critical to our objectives.

Strength and conditioning training is a process that breaks down current muscles to build new ones. And stronger muscles are built during recovery. How then will the body create newer muscles from nothing? First, you must feed it with proper nutrients to make gains. Simply put, what and how much we eat is critical in S&C training.

Strength training or exercising without proper nutrition, especially not getting enough protein, can lead to loss of existing muscles. Moreover, if you are not eating a balanced diet, you most likely won't have enough energy to exercise in the first place.

As you can see, S&C training is a gradual process and one that requires some effort. The practice is not something that can give us overnight results. It will take a little time to become stronger, have better balance, and have more energy. But, we can achieve our objectives much faster with proper nutrition.

To gain muscles and build strength with our eating, we must.

- Hydrate
- Take in enough calories
- Add enough protein to rebuild lost tissue

HYDRATION

"Water is the most neglected nutrient in your diet, but one of the most vital." – Julia Child

Hydration is the body's potential to take in water for daily use based on availability. Our cells, tissues, muscles, and organs need fluid to perform their functions efficiently. We need water to lubricate our joints, remove wastes, regulate our temperature, keep infections at bay, transport oxygen and nutrients to cells and tissues and maintain organ functionality. Studies also show that proper hydration improves mood, sleep quality, and cognition.

Liquids, particularly water, provide most of the fluid necessary for normal body function, but the food we consume provides up to 20% of our daily water intake. Many nutrition experts, talk show hosts, and magazines are now obsessed with the idea of "8 glasses daily." But, how much water should we actually take in to stay hydrated?

First, to stay "hydrated" means providing your body with enough fluids for ultimate functionality. The American Heart Association reports that fluid requirements vary significantly from one person to the next. A simple way to test whether you are well-hydrated is by checking your urine. You are dehydrated if it has a brown hue and well-hydrated if it is pale.

Remember that normal body functions such as urination, sweating, and breathing use the water in our body. Therefore, we must replace the water we lose frequently. The amount of water our bodies need may be affected by factors like exercise, age, climate, and diet.

Experts recommend around 6-11 glasses of water every day. Others recommend taking at least 1/3 of our total body weight in fluids. For example, suppose you weigh 210 pounds; your daily water intake goal should be at least 70 ounces of water. These numbers are not one-size-fits-all situations because, as mentioned above, everyone's water requirement is different. While plain water is the primary hydration source, we can supplement our intake with fruit-flavored water, fresh juice, etc. We should also adjust our consumption levels depending on the weather, illness, and daily activities such as training.

Sugar-sweetened drinks, including tea and coffee, don't do much for your hydration. In fact, drinks with caffeine have the opposite effect. Consider staying away from those if you struggle with staying hydrated. Studies show that Americans are pretty obsessed with sweetened foods and drinks. Most of us expect sugar in everything we consume, whether conscious of it or not. As a result, we take in so many sweetened beverages, most of which do nothing for our health.

Even the "innocent-looking" flavored and vitamin waters are loaded with unnecessary sugar. So, it's always a good rule of thumb to check the ingredients on the label before consuming. Studies show that vitamin and flavored water are no better. They are just as crummy as any other sugary beverage. These kinds of drinks are also strongly linked to obesity and weight gain.

If you trust marketing labels such as "B-vitamins," "electrolytes," or "zinc," and the more attractive phrases like "energy" or "revival," then you are in for a big surprise. Some of these drinks will power you up, but at a cost to your health.

We've all fallen at some point for the tempting labeling lingo. It's often convincing yet confusing, and we can barely differentiate snakeskin oil from plain water these days. The empty promises of food touted as "health food" have lined our shelves for too long. But with all the recent research, we should no longer fall for these flashy marketing strategies. So please read through the ingredients carefully before grabbing a "revitalizing" bottle of water.

Dehydration

When we neglect our body's fluid needs, we may become dehydrated. Illness can also cause dehydration, especially where there is vomiting and diarrhea. Considering how important water is to our overall health, it is understandable that studies show the effects of dehydration to be wide-ranging in severity and nature.

On one side, dehydration can cause headaches, dizziness, thirst, and lethargy. These don't sound significant until you learn that dehydration is a serious condition that can be life-threatening. Going for too long without enough water will cause our bodies to shut down, including kidney failure and brain swelling.

As the body struggles with dehydration, the heart rate gradually increases to compensate for insufficient fluid in the blood. Slowly, the most critical body organs like the lungs and brain don't receive the available fluids. Acute kidney injury (AKI) is a severe yet common dehydration-related condition. AKI is directly linked to reduced blood flow to the kidneys and affects recurrent dehydration.

Other common problems associated with dehydration include blood-clot-related complications, UTIs, heart problems, and even stroke. As you can imagine, dehydration affects our cells and tissues directly, and our immunity may suffer, so our bodies can't fight off infection and rebuild new tissue after injury.

Old age aggravates dehydration-related issues, too, so we must maintain the proper water intake in our senior years. Sadly, up to 40% of seniors could be chronically dehydrated, according to a recent study from the University of California.

As we age, our appetites and thirst levels start to decline. And when our body is deprived of necessary fluids, it may go unnoticed because we might be completely unaware. Dehydration can sneak up on us because it's not something we can automatically sense until we're already dehydrated.

Things that can cause dehydration:

- Thirst levels decline with age
- Decline in internal temperature regulation abilities
- Changes in body composition
- Underlying medical issues
- Certain medications used to treat these underlying issues
- Heat exposure

NUTRITION IN OLDER ADULTS

Why should we care about proper nutrition when modern medicine significantly increases our life expectancy? Well, the goal isn't just the length of life but the quality of life lived in those extra years. Long life is good, but not if we spend it in and out of hospital beds. Therefore, we must strive for a better quality of life for as long as we can still have it. Isn't it every senior's dream to enjoy retirement, have fun traveling the world, run after grandkids, and enjoy a fulfilling life without the torture of constant aches and pains?

Nutrition improves our lifespan and our general quality of life. And while it's good to start this mindset when we're young, striving for excellent nutrition can make a significant difference even after we are old, aches, pains, and all. This isn't to say that we'll become a new breed of ageless superhumans, but it can allow us to age gracefully and improve our resilience.

Many people have amazing bodies at 20 – athletic, slim, powerful even. However, by 70, seniors will have issues related to joint pain, blood sugar, pressure, and heart health, among other things. While many of us refer to these changes as "old age," "aging," etc., studies show that most of these things are an accumulation of lifestyle habits over many decades.

Other studies have shown that nutritional needs increase with age, even as our need for calories decreases. So now more than ever, seniors need a nutrient-dense, well-supplemented menu. And it doesn't have to be a lengthy, complicated process. It can and should be pretty straightforward.

The *Dietary Guidelines for Americans* recommends the following food groups to help seniors with their nutritional needs as they age:

Vegetables and Fruits

Fruits and vegetables are nutritious, whether fresh, canned, or frozen. Dark green vegetables like kale or broccoli are the best. Orange vegetables, including pumpkins, carrots, and butternut squash, are also highly beneficial for us.

Proteins

Foods like beans, peas, fish, eggs, meat, and milk can provide various necessary proteins.

Cereals

Go for whole grains where possible. Our bodies need at least three ounces of whole grain daily. Whole grains could be rice, cereals, bread, etc.

Milk, cheese, or yogurt

Our bodies need vitamin D to keep our bones strong and healthy. Take at least three servings of low or fat-free dairy products daily. There are also all kinds of non-dairy milk like almond, coconut, and oat milk that are fantastic sources of nutrients, too…and some of them taste amazing.

Fats

Prepare your food with oils and not solid fat. The fat should be monounsaturated (good fat) or polyunsaturated. Fish, certain vegetable oils, and nuts can be good sources of fats.

Techniques to help with nutrition

Consume whole foods. They have more nutrients and will improve overall nutrition.

Food supplements are also helpful. For example, you can incorporate natural protein shakes, fish oils, or fiber powders to increase and "supplement" nutrition.

Fruit smoothies are a great meal replacement and allow for incredible creativity. As a family, we make smoothies at least once a week as they can be a quick and nutritious solution filled with protein, complex carbohydrates, and good fats.

Ensure the meals are balanced; proteins, veggies, carbs, and fats.

If you can afford it, try a grocery delivery service to cut on time spent on food preparation.

Choose foods that are easy to prepare, like pre-made soups or proteins, fresh, pre-cut fruits, and vegetables.

This technique isn't for everyone, but try blending soft and well-cooked foods like mashed potatoes, scrambled eggs, soups, etc., that are easy to digest. It will certainly taste different than if eaten separately, but it will retain the necessary nutrients.

COMPONENTS OF GOOD NUTRITION FOR SENIORS

Our bodies need good nutrition to manage rigorous training, endure and recover from it and build strength.

Our body needs amino acids to rebuild stronger muscles and build strength, especially after weightlifting and exercises. Amino acids come from beef, eggs, poultry, fish, beans, legumes, etc.

Calcium is stored in bones and maintains muscle health. Without calcium, our bones will become fragile and slowly start to decay. Whole grains, leafy greens, and dairy products are excellent sources of calcium.

Fats surround our cells, so we must consume them in small quantities. It's healthier to choose monounsaturated fats over saturated fat.

What is it about pepper that makes them hot? What about ginger, cinnamon, or even carrots give those distinctive colors and tastes? Well, phytochemicals are responsible for this. Phytochemicals are the complex compounds in vegetables, fruits, and other plants that give them their colors, aroma, and flavors. They are powerful and complex, so you'll never confuse a clove of garlic with a piece of ginger root.

Phytochemicals are well-known sources of anti-inflammatory, antioxidant, and antihistamine agents. These agents are crucial for injury recovery following exercise. In addition, phytochemicals can revive our immune system, slow down the growth of cancerous cells and maintain our DNA's health and general health. Colorful vegetables and fruits provide us with enough phytochemicals, which is why doctors and nutritionists encourage us to eat balanced diets, which include seeds, nuts, legumes, vegetables, fruits, etc.

To fight free radicals, we need antioxidants, primarily found in fruits and vegetables. Antioxidants are powerful, helping us rid our bodies of toxins, pollution, and cancerous cells.

Vitamins and minerals help us process everything that goes through our system and keeps the body working in excellent conditions. Fruits, vegetables, and certain whole-grain cereals often contain the best vitamins and minerals.

Protein, Fat, Carb Intake: What is Recommended?

Research shows that seniors need more protein. A PROT-AGE Study group 2, released in 2013, recommends at least 1-1.2 grams of proteins for every 1 kilogram of body weight. The European Society for Clinical Nutrition and Metabolism (ESPEN) echoed the same protein recommendations for seniors.

While additional research is still needed to establish the exact facts relating to daily protein intake for seniors, expert opinion suggests 1-1.2 grams of protein/kg for muscle preservation. For example, a senior weighing 150 pounds needs between 60-80 grams of protein daily.

To calculate your approximate daily protein intake, convert your weight into kilograms by dividing it by 2.2, then multiply that figure by 0.8. We may even need more protein in certain circumstances, such as when we are in the hospital recovering from injury or when there is a non-healing wound or pressure injury. On the other hand, a senior may sometimes need less protein when dealing with kidney disease.

The United States Department of Agriculture recommends healthier protein options such as lentils, seafood, and beans over red meat to minimize the risk of heart conditions while providing the body with enough protein for normal bodily functions. That's because beans and lentils are more nutrient-dense than red meat. Yes, they have fewer fats and calories, but they provide more vitamins, minerals, and proteins for the same amount of red meat.

If you eat 100g of lentils, you already have 32% of the daily required fiber in your system. As a result, you'll feel fuller for longer and lower your risk of heart-related issues. Beef provides no fiber and more of the less recommended saturated fat. On the contrary, lentils provide no vitamin B-12, while beef provides more vitamin B-12, niacin, vitamin B-6, riboflavin, and sodium.

Red meat is okay, but not regularly; even then, it should be in small amounts. You should eat red meat to acquire the vitamins not contained in cereals, but it's best to stick to lean beef and avoid too many processed types of meat like sausages, salami, hotdogs, etc.

Fats

The USDA recommends around 20-35% of a senior adult's daily calorie intake should be fat. Saturated fats should make less than 10% of the overall fat given the calorie intake. Saturated fats are the unhealthier type, usually solid at room temperature, and primarily found in animal products such as dairy and red meat. Too much saturated fat raises our bad cholesterol levels.

The average recommended fat intake is no more than 30g for the average man and no more than 20g for the average woman. Better yet, we can replace saturated fat with unsaturated fat - those that are liquid at room temperature.

Please remember that heart disease is linked to other factors, including lifestyle habits, and is not limited to diet only.

Carbohydrates

The National Institute of Aging recommends around 45-65% of the total daily calorie intake in a senior adult's diet be carbohydrates.

A higher percentage of these carbohydrates should be starchy vegetables, complex carbs, legumes, or whole grains. Complex carbohydrates like sweet potatoes keep older adults in the healthy blood sugar range, even as glucose tolerance reduces over the years.

As stated by the National Institute of Aging (NIA), we need more fibers in the diet in our senior years. Fiber improves bowel movements while reducing the risk of heart disease and diabetes. Thirty grams of fiber per day is recommended for men, while females should aim for 20-25 grams daily.

Good sources of fiber include:

- Vegetables
- Fruits
- Grains
- Nuts and seeds

- Legumes
- Whole-grain products such as corn, brown rice, barley, wild rice, etc.

What is "quality protein"?

Many of us are only familiar with proteins, their sources, and how they contribute to overall health. Some people may not know that protein quality matters too, and it is more important than quantity.

But what is protein quality?

How well can a particular protein perform the metabolic functions expected in the body? Quality proteins perform their metabolic functions well; the opposite is true of poor-quality proteins. So how is protein quality tested? By 1. Its digestibility, 2. The potential supply of all the necessary amino acids needed for normal body functions.

Quality proteins have a high digestible value, meaning the body can easily break them down and use them for normal body functions. They also have a higher biological value, which is the quality they offer. Quality proteins provide all the necessary amino acids required by the body.

Quality proteins are essential because they form the basis of muscle formation, which is very important in S&C training. Eating high-quality proteins after some rigorous exercises helps the body repair any kind of damage done to muscle fibers. Always go for the healthiest option available: plant or animal-based protein.

High-quality proteins

- Animal products such as meat, fish, poultry, and dairy products
- Fish such as salmon, tuna, and whitefish
- Eggs
- Quinoa is a high-quality plant-based protein
- Soy such as Tofu and edameme
- Lentils
- Whey

Low-quality proteins

- Bread or other cereal-based products
- Nut butter such as cashew, peanut, and almond
- Seeds such as pumpkin, sunflower, chia, and hemp

We should consume high-quality proteins or at least a few of these to obtain the amino acids for normal body function.

Sugar: The Antihero

The antihero in a play or movie is usually a character who is neither completely bad nor completely good. In some cases, they may lack a particular moral compass and traditional attributes that you'd see in the typical hero who "saves the day." Yet, we often find ourselves rooting for antiheroes because they can be very relatable and attractive. Such is the case with sugar.

While it's true that sugar occurs naturally in all starchy foods, including grains, vegetables, and fruits, it is the healthy type, providing the body with a steady supply of energy throughout the day. Processed sugar, on the other hand, has a bad reputation. Refined sugar is directly linked to an increased risk of cardiovascular disease, as the Journal of the American Medical Association reported. So sugar presents us with a dichotomy, a split personality. It's the antihero.

The risk of heart disease more than doubles in individuals whose sugar intake is equal to or more than 21% of their daily calorie intake. So, if an average American man consumes up to 24 teaspoons of refined sugar, equivalent to 384 calories every day, they are much more at risk of predisposing themselves to cardiovascular disease.

Consumption of refined sugar has tripled worldwide over the last five decades. Unfortunately, the American diet is a big offender in the refined sugar discussion. You can find refined sugar in many processed foods, soft drinks, baked foods, yogurt, and other "innocent" foods, including soups, ketchup, bread, etc.

So, how much sugar should we eat?

First, understand that sugar is not a nutritional requirement, particularly refined sugar. For this reason, it's hard to give it an absolute figure. According to the American Heart Association, women should consume no more than 24 grams/6 teaspoons/100 calories of sugar daily, while men shouldn't take more than 36 grams/9 teaspoons/150 calories daily.

While natural sugar has some benefits, research has linked added sugar to:

- Diabetes – consuming large amounts of added sugar leads to weight gain, which increases the risk of diseases, including diabetes and heart disease.
- Cancer – studies have revealed that added sugar increases cancer risk, including colon, breast, esophageal, and intestinal cancer.
- Gut leakage – excess sugar can cause inflammation which may result in leakage of contents from the intestines to the bloodstream.
- Nonalcoholic fatty liver disease – this liver condition is linked to obesity, diabetes, and insulin resistance, which are directly associated with excess sugar.
- Liver failure – sugar worsens inflammation, which can lead to complete shutdown.

So, how can we minimize added sugar?

The first step is awareness. For example, added sugar isn't always referred to as "sugar"; it exists in many forms under different names. If you spot the following terms as an ingredient in a particular product, cut back on the frequency of consumption or avoid it altogether.

- Molasses
- Honey
- Nectars
- Sugar, brown sugar, raw sugar, white granulated sugar, and inverted sugar.
- Dextrose, fructose, lactose, sucrose, maltose
- Syrup, malt syrup, corn syrup, pancake syrup, high-fructose corn syrup
- Corn sweetener
- Fruit juice concentrates
- Liquid sugar, powder sugar, sugar cubes
- Artificial sweeteners like sucralose, xylitol, mannitol, and sorbitol

The amount of sugar in a product is often listed as "total sugar" and is measured in grams. Look out for the total number of servings and grams in each product. The listing may only show 5 grams, but there could be five servings of the given product. So, you could easily consume 20 grams of sugar without even noticing.

Track the amount of sugar consumed in your beverages too. A 2017 Public Health study reports that the general population consumes nearly half of all added sugar in drinks like coffee and tea. More than two-thirds of coffee drinkers and a third of tea drinkers use refined sugar in one form or another. If more than 60% of the calories consumed in beverages come from added sugar, then it's time to rethink the nutritional benefits of these drinks we crave.

If you have a choice (and we do), why not just avoid these beverages altogether? I know this can be tough because I personally love coffee and tea. My coffee additives are usually a few heaping tablespoons of half-and-half and an occasional splash of chocolate almond milk. And I often put a large tablespoon (or two) of honey into my earl grey tea. We all have our vices, yes? But what are some healthy alternatives that might give us some balanced options?

Given the seemingly endless list of sugar variations we should avoid, we should investigate some healthier alternatives. Believe it or not, the list of healthy options is pretty robust, so have hope. Keep in mind that while these alternatives still contain sugar, they can be quickly metabolized and offer a higher nutritional value than added sugar. These are:

- Honey
- Maple syrup
- Coconut sugar
- Jaggery

The Upside of Sugar

Without sugar, life (and diet) would be incomplete because we do still need it in healthy doses.

Sugar improves brain function.

Sugar is a powerful mood booster, which is why most people crave it when they feel low. By giving them the proper energy, sugar boosts our brain cells and spurs them into action.

Sugar is also an excellent source of energy.

Adding those extra calories to tea or coffee jumpstarts your day, giving you the energy to start your day on a positive high.

Sugar is also a natural source of glycolic acid, a compound that protects the skin from harmful UV rays, premature aging, and sun damage. As a result, sugar is an effective DIY skin and lip scrub. You don't have to spend thousands at the spa when you can easily make a simple homemade scrub using the sugar already available in your kitchen.

It's obvious which list is longer, but sugar is not entirely the bad guy we should completely malign regarding our health. When consumed moderately, sugar can perform excellent functions within our bodies. It's the perfect antihero.

Whole Foods vs. Processed Foods. Which is better?

Before diving into the conversation about which is better, we must first understand the difference between processed and whole foods.

In the simplest definition, "processed" in this case refers to any food whose natural state has been altered through processing, the addition of extra ingredients, sugar, salt, preservatives, etc.

Whole foods have undergone none of the processes mentioned above. Most are still in their natural state or as close to it as possible. Whole foods are calorie-dense and usually get digested over a long period, and these foods continuously provide the body with energy, making them the healthiest option.

Examples of whole foods

- Fresh meat and seafood with no additives
- Fresh fruits, vegetables, and herbs
- Fresh and dry beans
- Lentils
- Grains
- Nuts and seeds

Not all processing is "bad" because when we go deeper into this conversation, we realize that minimally processed foods, like grilled chicken breast, are considered "processed" but are still as nutritious and healthy as some whole foods. Certain foods must be "processed" to a certain degree to be considered edible in the first place. So the only difference is in the amount of processing.

Minimally processed foods have undergone a single step or very few steps of processing. A few of these may have had minor things added and may contain some mild preservatives. Examples of these are:

- Whole grain products such as bread
- Snacks packaged with nothing other than salt/sugar/oil
- Cheese
- Yogurt
- Pasteurized products like milk – particularly plant-based
- Canned products including vegetables, fruits
- Jarred vegetables
- Dried, frozen, smoked products
- Sauces and dressings
- Jams, jellies, and butter
- Dried, frozen

Even when marketed as "low calorie/fat," processed foods can still negatively impact our health, which is the exact opposite of what processed foods marketing campaigns imply.

We also have ultra-processed foods, which have gone through multiple processes before being sold off as finished products. Most ultra-processed foods add little to no nutritional value; they are highly addictive and even delicious to a certain degree. They have high quantities of refined carbs, fats, sodium, sugar, and other unhealthy additives. Ultra-processed foods are the types of food that will first come into your mind when you think of "processed" foods.

Examples of ultra-processed foods:

- Frozen pizza
- Baked foods like cookies, cakes, bread, crackers, etc.
- Soft drinks like sodas and sweetened beverages
- Snacks, sweets,
- Ready-made cereals
- Meat-like products – hot dogs, sausages, etc.

- Chicken nuggets, burgers, fries

Unlike sugar, we should avoid ultra-processed foods at all costs. All they do is contribute to the glucose spike in the body and nothing more.

The National Institute of Health did a recent study comparing the impact of ultra-processed versus whole foods, revealing some eye-opening details. For example, when put on a processed foods diet, healthy adults gained up to one pound weekly. However, when placed on whole-food diets, they lost weight. Maybe you expected this.

But you might not have expected that weight differences existed even though the two diets' caloric values were the same. This means that even when you eat an equal number of calories in ultra-processed foods as you would whole foods, you will probably gain weight. Furthermore, the study shows that, on average, people on the ultra-processed diet generally ate more calories but ate less when on the whole foods diet.

Why are whole foods better?

Whole foods have a wide variety of nutritional benefits.

They have more fiber and fewer fats.

If we want to reduce the bad fats (trans and saturated fats) and increase our intake of good fats (omega or monounsaturated fats), we should eat more whole foods. Because they have more fiber, whole foods improve bowel movement and keep the GI tract in motion. As a result, we'll feel fuller faster and less likely to overeat.

Because the body breaks them down slowly, we are also less likely to have glucose spikes, reducing the risk of blood sugar.

Whole foods reduce the risk of inflammation.

Inflammation is linked directly to arthritis, high blood sugar, cancer, and heart disease. Whole foods digest slowly, which means the natural sugars contained in them are not released in large enough amounts to cause inflammation, unlike ultra-processed foods.

Balance is critical when it comes to processed and whole foods. We don't have to completely cut out processed foods from our diet, but we should know where to draw the line. Practice moderation with your diet, just like all other things in life. But, if we're able, we should still try to avoid the unhealthier alternatives altogether.

Lean Muscle Foods.

How much would you weigh if you had no fat in your body? Think bones, skin, ligaments, tendons, and body water. Would you weigh a little or a lot? That's your lean body mass. So, have you guessed what lean muscle mass is, following the definition of lean body mass? Lean muscle is the percentage of muscle composition in your body.

At a glance, two people may look or even weigh the same. However, if the muscle composition of each individual was to be analyzed, you may find that one has a higher muscle mass than the other. So why is lean muscle important, especially in older adults?

Lean muscle has a direct impact on lean body mass. It's essential to look and feel great, toned, strong, and muscular, but it's more than that. To build a healthy body long-term, we must first build on lean muscles.

Studies show that a higher lean muscle and body mass protects our bones as we age, protecting them against thinning and weakening. As we know, osteoporosis is a real danger as we age. The frailty that comes with age also increases the risk of falls and fractures. For this reason, experts recommend optimizing muscle mass to improve bone density and strength.

Our lean body mass affects our basal metabolic rate (BMR) – the number of calories burned at rest. Therefore, the higher the percentage of lean body mass there is, the more calories can burn while resting. Simply put, if you have a higher lean body mass, you burn more calories, which helps reduce the risk of obesity that is usually associated with calorie imbalances.

By now, you know that we lose muscle mass as we age, a condition known as sarcopenia in the medical field. Sarcopenia affects mobility, muscle strength, and the overall ability to be independent. And that's without mentioning the improved risk of frailty, fall and fracture-related disabilities, depression, and the subsequent loss of independence.

Consequently, we must ask ourselves how we can build lean muscles or prevent the loss of what we already have if we are to maintain our health in later years.

So, how can we improve lean muscle?

Diet, physical activity, and movement are critical in building lean muscle, which is why you are reading about it in a strength and conditioning book. However, while it's important to challenge ourselves through exercise, we must also build on our nutritional requirements. To gain muscle, we must stack up on protein-rich foods and add fats and carbohydrates, so we have enough energy to train.

Which foods help build lean muscles? Protein-rich foods like:

- Eggs
- Fish including salmon, tuna, and tilapia
- Chicken, Turkey
- Lean red meat, including beef, lamb, and bison
- Shrimp
- Beans, Lentils
- Protein shakes
- Milk and dairy products

- Bison
- Quinoa
- Nuts
- Chickpeas, among others

The strengths and weaknesses of a plant-based diet

As the name suggests, a plant-based diet focuses on plant produce like fruits, vegetables, nuts, and grains with little-to-no animal products like eggs, milk, and meat. People opt for plant-based diets for many reasons, including animal welfare, environmental benefits, health benefits, and personal preference. While it's true that plant-based diets can reduce the risk of heart disease and support all our nutritional needs, we must tread this path carefully and plan these diets well.

There are many plant-based diets, so everyone can choose what works for them if they decide to go down this path.

- Vegans: Don't consume animal-based products, including eggs, dairy, or honey.
- Semi-vegetarians: Have limited their intake of dairy, eggs, seafood, poultry, and meat options. However, they may opt for one or eat them occasionally.
- Ovo-vegetarians: Eat eggs and no other animal-related produce, including dairy.
- Lacto vegetarians: Eat only dairy foods but not meat, eggs, seafood, or poultry.
- Lacto-Ovo vegetarians: They eat eggs and dairy, excluding seafood, poultry, and meat.
- Pescatarians: Eat shellfish and fish only.
- Pegans: This is a relatively new diet. It's pronounced like Vegans, but with a "P." The Pegan diet combines paleo (fruits, nuts, eggs, wild meat) and vegan foods.

While plant-based diets offer affordable, nutritious, and tasty alternatives, they don't readily provide enough vitamin B12, which can pose a dilemma for those who are 100% vegans. You can find B12 in seaweed (nori), shitake mushrooms, and nutritional yeast, but that's about it.

Pros of plant-based diets

Research backs up plant-based diets as a powerful force in improving health outcomes.

- It improves our cardiovascular health by reducing blood pressure and heart rate.
- Reduces the levels of bad cholesterol while raising the levels of good cholesterol in the bloodstream.
- Significantly reduced the risk of diabetes, particularly type II.
- It is directly linked to improved cognitive function, delaying the onset and even minimizing the symptoms of Alzheimer's and dementia.
- Reduces the risk of obesity and correlated conditions.

Cons of plant-based diets

A plant-based diet is a good thing and guaranteed to improve our health significantly. However, this diet needs proper planning and a conscious balance of the foods eaten. So, it's not something you approach blindly, and it's not for everybody.

Some health concerns to look out for include:

- Iron deficiency
- Deficiency of vitamin B12
- Increased risk of fractures from calcium and vitamin D deficiency
- Reduced protein intake
- Deficiency in essential fatty and amino acids

The general concept of a plant-based diet is shifting towards a more flexible approach. Many people are adopting an individualized approach that is healthier and nutritious. If you need vitamin B12, iron, more protein, or calcium, you'd have to be flexible even if you are being environmentally cautious and adopting healthier options.

Please be mindful that if you're considering a new diet plan (like the ones above), it's always a good idea to chat with a local health professional before you alter your meals. Ask your doctor, a nutritionist, or a registered dietitian to help you create a game plan to find the best nutritional options that work for you.

Breakfast. Is it the most important meal of the day?

But why? Why is breakfast the most necessary meal of the day?

There are many good reasons, backed by research and many studies. Breakfast is the lead-off meal of the day after a long period of overnight "fasting." Breakfast spurs our metabolism into action, providing us with enough glucose to renew our energy and boost our mental alertness.

Good research has highlighted the numerous benefits of breakfast, including improved health, memory, and metabolism, which reduces the risk of heart disease, diabetes, and obesity.

There is one thing many experts agree on, skipping breakfast can throw you off. Remember, by being asleep, you obviously won't be eating anything, so when you wake up, the blood sugar needed to kick-start your muscles and brain will be at an all-time low. Breakfast is the trick. It is what replenishes our body and prepares it for the day. If the body gets deprived of this morning boost or glucose, we may feel less energetic as we go about our day. To compensate for this, we may overeat when we finally decide to eat.

Breakfast also allows us to eat some vitamins, proteins, and other nutrients by eating grains, dairy, and fruits.

It's unfortunate then that many people skip breakfast because they are in a hurry to get out of the house. It shouldn't be this way because there are many efficient ways to make breakfast. Your system really needs food sooner than lunchtime.

Several studies report that people who eat a healthy breakfast have a thinner waistline than those who don't. But how can this be? Proteins and fiber keep you fuller for longer. Eating a protein-rich breakfast keeps your appetite in check throughout the day. Skipping a meal doesn't help with weight loss, even if you are on a diet.

Eating breakfast while on a diet will do you good because you are less likely to overeat during the day. And it would be best if you resisted the temptation to grab those cakes and donuts from your favorite shop. A balanced breakfast should contain fiber, protein, carbohydrates, fats, and even grains. Fiber keeps you full throughout the day, carbohydrates provide the glucose to boost your energy and brain activity, and proteins will provide the energy needed a few hours from now.

And if you've heard people repeating the old phrase, *"Eat breakfast like a king, eat lunch like a prince, and eat dinner like a pauper,"* you'd understand if I told you that yesterday's leftovers are even better. So warm them quickly and kick off your morning metabolism with a healthy dose of energy.

Beyond leftovers, some other healthy options for breakfast include – smoothies, eggs, oatmeal, or whole-grain cereals made with low-fat milk or yogurt, fruits, and nuts.

Chapter 6

Well Oiled Machine: Pre, Workout, Post

"Give me six hours to chop down a tree, and I will spend the first four sharpening the ax."

- Abraham Lincoln, 16th President of the USA

Preparation is undoubtedly the key to being successful in anything, and there is no exception when building more strength and better conditioning. Preparing or what I like to call "ramping up" to the three phases of our workouts helps us prepare for the stress on the mind and body that lie ahead. If we've well prepared, we can almost guarantee that we'll perform our workouts at a higher level of intensity.

Ramping up isn't difficult. It's really about getting into the right mindset to perform the workouts. When done enough times, it starts to become routine. Ramping up is just creating simple habits or techniques to prepare you. For those who have worked out, these are already part of our fitness DNA in some shape or form. For those who haven't, it may take a little time for these to become routine for you. But don't worry. These can quickly assimilate into your daily routine after a bit of practice.

Developing simple "ramping up" techniques has numerous strategic benefits. They can affect physical things like reducing our risk of injury. And they help our mental focus by boosting our confidence. So here are some simple techniques that will get you rolling in the right direction without even breaking a sweat.

- Focus on better breathing - Take five deep breaths when you get up in the morning. Breathing exercises stimulate the body by increasing the amount of oxygen in the bloodstream, making us feel more alert. Sometimes closing your eyes and blocking out all distractions while breathing helps this moment become more effective. As brief as this technique is, it can help center you before starting your day.
- Another technique is visualization - For example, try visualizing what a typical day will look like for you. Then you could make a simple mental note about a new exercise or stretch that you want to try or set a new nutritional goal for that day. This technique compliments the morning breathing routine.

- Increase water intake - Drinking a glass of water (or more) every morning has many benefits. It hydrates your body, lowers your calorie intake, aids weight reduction, boosts mental function, promotes skin health, and kick-starts your metabolism.
- Body mechanics awareness - Other pre-workout strategies include basic movement awareness, light stretching, and moderate bending and reaching. This might sound silly, but try being conscious of your body mechanics during simple tasks like opening a kitchen cupboard, folding a shirt, or getting almond milk from the fridge. This technique can help prepare your mind for workouts by making you more aware of how your body works. You can accentuate the motions slowly and make them into a stretch, bend or reach technique. And this is why we exercise, right…to ensure our bodies work well for our daily tasks.

PHASE 1: PRE-WORKOUT

Preparing the Body

If you've exercised before, you are probably guilty of jumping into a workout without a good warm-up. I know I am. We often become hasty for results and want to dive into the nuts and bolts of the exercise. Consequently, we might do some quick stretching and maybe a light jog, if anything. And then we wonder why we end up stiff and sore the next day instead of loose and limber. These hasty preparations might help start our heart rate going a bit, and it's better than nothing. But it's not an excellent long-term approach to prepare the body every time we exercise.

The pre-workout phase is arguably an essential part of any workout. It's the phase before our body puts all the tools in place to perform optimally during each specific exercise. If we don't correctly warm up, we will set ourselves up for potential injuries and performance setbacks. Therefore this step, the pre-workout, is so important.

This phase aims to get the blood flowing and prepping your body for exercise. We do this through light cardio activity (like walking in place) or a warm-up routine that specifically addresses the muscle group you're addressing during your workout. A good example would be a warm-up routine for legs that stretches out all the muscles used during squats or lunges, especially quads and hamstrings, which have tendons that stretch throughout the day and need extra attention before exercise.

According to studies, the pre-workout phase is also critical for muscle repair and growth. Without it, our bodies can't generate optimal energy for training, leading to an ineffective workout and potentially overtraining syndrome (a condition that occurs when you train too hard beyond the limits without giving your body enough time to rest.)

Whether you're in the mood for a high-intensity custom workout (see Chapter 9) or a low-key walk around the neighborhood, it's essential to take care of your body with a pre-workout routine before you begin.

The following are some helpful tips on preparing your body, so you can get out there and enjoy the benefits and reap the rewards of working out!

Nutrition

Make sure your body has energy before you begin. As mentioned in Chapter 5, a good breakfast and hydration are essential to fuel our muscles throughout the day. Nutrition is also critical after your workout, which we'll review soon.

Here are some key benefits of proper nutrition relating to pre-workouts:

Carbohydrates: Carbohydrates provide energy to your muscles. This energy (glucose) is stored in the liver and muscles as glycogen. Numerous studies show that carbs promote glycogen storage and utilization. They help our muscles get more prepared for the oncoming exercise and keep them fresh and at their highest level of performance.

Proteins: Eating foods high in protein slows down digestion and prolongs the feeling of satiety. Eating protein-rich foods during the pre-workout phase reduces hunger cravings and prevents overeating. Protein is one of the most crucial building blocks for working out as it helps your muscles recover and repair faster.

Fats: Recent research has shown that consuming food rich in fats one hour before working out can increase the activity of your muscle cells.

To maximize nutritional benefits before you work out, you should eat a meal rich in fats. Here are three reasons why:

1. Fat provides the most energy per gram than carbohydrates and protein. Thus, it fuels your muscles more during the workout.
2. Fats help release insulin from your pancreas to shuttle amino acids (protein building blocks) into muscle cells, helping them grow bigger and stronger so you can build lean muscle mass.
3. Since insulin also carries potassium into muscle cells, your body has more energy to work out longer and harder.

Examples of good fats to eat for pre-workout

- Nuts and seeds
- Avocados
- Chicken and turkey
- Egg whites

Water

Drink water prior to, during, and after your workout. Water helps improve our circulation, which improves oxygen flow and transportation of nutrients to our muscles. When these are optimal, our body can perform all its functions more efficiently during exercise.

Stretching, Warming up

We will cover specific stretches for each body part in Chapter 8, but I want to note that we need to warm up the body and adequately stretch before any workout.

Here are the benefits of stretching:

- Stimulates and lubricates joints: All joints have synovial fluid that acts as a lubricant. We can compare its viscosity to that of honey. Our joints are sometimes stiff when we wake up because the synovial fluid is thick. As we warm up, the fluid's viscosity decreases, becoming water-thin. This process makes our joints more mobile and less stiff.
- Increases temperature and blood flow to tissues: Exercising muscles generates heat, which your body regulates through thermoregulation. The more active and functioning a muscle is, the more blood gets transported to it to provide nutrients and oxygen.
- Enhances neuromuscular coordination: Stretching increases neuromuscular coordination. It improves how our muscles, bones, and joints work together. The more we do it, the more efficient we become at making things work smoothly together.

Additionally, when bones, muscles, joints, and nerves are efficient, they need less energy to function correctly, which means it takes less physical effort to complete specific movements. And that means you can exercise more with less effort, making it easier to move the body's mass.

Warming up also increases the speed at which your brain can send signals through your body. For example, when you're lifting weights, your muscles need to be contracted to lift the weights. More efficient muscle contraction means better coordination between your brain and the muscles.

While stretching is crucial for our workouts, there are some Dos and Don'ts to keep in mind:

Stretching Do's

- Do regular stretching. For long-term results, perform daily stretches and be consistent.
- Warm-up time should be around 5-10; however, this varies depending on age, exercise frequency, and physical condition.
- Focus on general muscle groups (neck, shoulders, chest, etc.) and the individual muscles therein.
- Break a little sweat. The idea is to heat our bodies to improve blood circulation. Mild intensity is good, but don't get too vigorous.
- Warm-up before or during stretching. To prevent tearing muscle fibers, we need to warm up before or as we stretch. When muscles and joints are warmed up, they loosen up and are less apt to get injured.

Stretching Don'ts

- Don't rush. We should never rush warm-ups and stretches; instead, we should do them slowly and carefully. The goal is to experience mild discomfort (in the muscles) rather than harsh agony.

- Don't warm up to the point of feeling pain; warm-ups should cause no pain. Stretching aims to prepare muscles and joints for a workout and speed up muscle recovery afterward.
- Don't forcefully twist your back - According to a 2018 study, low back pain is the top cause of disability worldwide. It may be tempting to stretch your back forcefully if it is stiff, but don't do it. So go easy when you stretch, especially with your back. The bones of our lower backs aren't built to rotate too much (not past 20 degrees).
- Don't stretch any injured body part.

Breathing, Visualization

As you stretch and warm up, start preparing your body with slightly deeper and slower breathing. As you're doing this, you can also begin visualizing your exercises, especially if you're just starting. Think about your form and posture from the start of the movement to the end.

Breathing, visualizing, and focusing on what you're doing before and during your workout can increase your chances of successful training. Proper breathing allows sufficient oxygenation of your muscles to work efficiently. In addition, it facilitates the aerobic mechanics of exercise and helps the body recover after an intense session.

Visualization is a great way to get into an exercise rhythm or groove. Finally, as we explained earlier, it will help focus your mind on your workout, ensuring you do everything as optimally as possible.

Visualizing your exercises from start to finish, especially when first starting out, can be very beneficial. Prepping your mind for what's about to take place can help maximize the success of your workout. This process includes seeing yourself performing each exercise perfectly from the first one to the last and even picturing yourself done, tired, and satisfied with your efforts. Granted, this does take a little extra time, but consider the benefits for your workouts and health.

While visualization helps us directly with our workouts, it can also help indirectly with:

- Boosting motivation
- Gaining confidence
- Relieving stress
- Improving mood
- Relieving pain
- Increasing muscle strength
- Speeding up healing

Lindsey Vonn and Visualization

Many of the most accomplished actors and decorated athletes regularly use visualization techniques before they perform. For example, Lindsey Vonn, one of the greatest Alpine skiers of all time, practiced visualization regularly. When Vonn finished competing in 2019, she disclosed one of her best-kept secrets. She revealed that her competitive edge was to visualize herself going down every course she competed on...hundreds of times. Vonn studied the courses extensively and said, "once I visualized a course, I'd never forget it ."Part of her visualization technique was putting specific body movements and breathing mechanics into every course turn, "I control my emotions and just make it routine." One can apply this technique to anything performance-related, especially strength and conditioning.

PHASE 2: THE WORKOUT

The Body During Exercise

This is where the rubber meets the road. We've prepared for this and are now ready to get down to business. In addition to the body mechanics of the exercises themselves, which we'll discuss in Chapters 9 and 10, there are a few things to remember when you work out. These are; breathing, form/posture, hydration, and patience.

Breathing

Good breathing is critical when we work out. First, it is imperative not to hold your breath during your workout repetitions. There may be a natural temptation to do this when first learning how to exercise. We often subconsciously think that holding our breath helps boost our strength. I see this a lot with beginners when they first start lifting weights. But surprisingly, the opposite is true. Instead, each exercise repetition (rep) should begin with an inhale before the rep starts. And as the rep starts, breathe out, ensuring exhalation is complete (when the rep ends). This breathing process will become second nature as you exercise.

Proper breathing provides a continuous flow of fresh air to the lungs, increasing stamina and endurance; it helps you inhale more oxygen, which is essential for burning body fat; and eliminating waste gasses from the body. After all, we do not want to feel out of breath while doing our exercises.

Other significant benefits of proper breathing include:

- Regulates blood pressure
- Strengthens the diaphragm
- Increases oxygen intake
- Improves endurance
- Strengthens muscles of the respiratory system

Hydration

Hydration is one of the most crucial facets of your workout, and how hydrated you are at the beginning of your exercise can dictate how well you perform. One effect of not being fully hydrated is the build-up of lactic acid in our bodies.

Lactic acid is a metabolic consequence that can lead to soreness and fatigue after your workout, often leading to increased recovery time. Lactic acid builds when there is a lack of oxygen in the body. The body cannot convert glucose into energy due to insufficient oxygen. As a result, something called lactate is produced to replace oxygen. So the best way to avoid this soreness is to stay hydrated.

Hydration increases the cardiovascular system's efficiency and blood flow to the muscles. When enough oxygen is in the body, it can efficiently metabolize lactic acid, thus reducing muscle fatigue and soreness. During a workout, it's essential to stay hydrated because we all lose water through sweat. Replenishing this water loss with adequate water consumption throughout your exercises will allow you to push harder and train longer.

Patience

Another essential element we need to remember while working out is patience. So many people become incredibly intolerant and want to get in shape as fast as possible. And I get it. We sometimes get unhappy with our shape, especially after the holidays. And we want to fast-track a solution to better bodies.

The problem with this approach is that it simply doesn't work long-term. Trying to lose weight in a short period by increasing the hours we exercise isn't a good idea, especially if you are starting to focus on changing your diet. You might lose some weight initially, but it won't help you develop good long-term habits. Instead, it would be best if you gave your body time to adjust to the new routines and learn how to exercise with weights correctly. Our family's motto is "slow and steady wins the race," and this phrase especially applies to strength and conditioning training.

Stay mindful as you approach your workouts that this is a long-term lifestyle change. You're trying to curb old habits and establish new ones. So keep a realistic mindset that you will learn and grow at this over time. Stay patient, stay consistent, and stay focused. Having unrealistic expectations and being hasty will set you up for disappointment.

PHASE 3: POST-WORKOUT

Recovery

The post-workout recovery period is almost as important as the workout itself, so allow yourself plenty of time to rest. Muscles need time to recoup and rebuild from the duress experienced during exercise. Often it takes hours or even days for muscles to heal, depending on how intense the workout is. Elite athletes frequently take days off specific body parts to recuperate from intense training. According to a published study in 2005 in the Journal of Applied Physiology, resting after a workout helps muscles rebuild much faster than if there's little or no rest.

Our bodies need rest to recuperate from and adapt to exercise. During training, we use our bodies energy stores, particularly carbohydrates (for energy) and fluids (lost through sweat). The body needs time to replenish these lost reserves. Multiple studies have highlighted the importance of rest; as it is, our bodies need at least 24 hours to replace their carbohydrate supply fully. As we know now, we must maintain muscle glycogen and the necessary sugar levels for energy.

Additionally, our bodies must replace lost fluids, which it does faster than carbohydrates. Research shows that one to two hours is usually enough for the body to recover from lost fluids. So we must give it at least that much time to do that.

As if that isn't enough, exercises may cause tissue damage. Some of the damage is beneficial because it leads to muscle growth, but other times, it's a painful nuisance. But if these muscles are to recover, scientifically known as physiological adaptation, they need periods of recovery and rest between exercises.

Many other adaptations our bodies undergo during and after exercise require rest and recovery. The quality of rest has also been a discussion in recent years. As it is, studies show that disturbed sleep patterns harm our performances and cognitive abilities significantly. I would encourage you to read articles about rest quality and its impact on exercise as it is impossible to cover everything I'd love to cover in a single book here.

Cool Down/Stretching

After a vigorous workout, it's essential to cool down and stretch out when your muscles are still warm and pliable. Cooling down can help your heart rate return to normal more quickly, preventing soreness, cramping, and injury. In addition, stretching helps to lengthen the muscle fibers and relieve tightness so that you can continue with other activities without experiencing any pain or discomfort.

Try doing 8-12 reps at a time of each stretch with about 30 seconds between each stretch. Doing this will help get the blood flowing back through your body and make you feel 100% after a great workout!

Nutrition

Post-workout nutrition is more important than one might think. Our bodies need the proper nutrients to repair themselves and recover from high-intensity training. For instance, protein helps repair muscle tissue, and carbohydrates replenish glucose stores that provide energy for your next workout.

A protein snack and hydration post-workout ensure your body replenishes the fuel you've just burned. In addition, hydrating after a workout will also help decrease muscle soreness from the build-up of lactic acid. During intense workouts, our bodies try hard to produce extra energy to sustain the activity through a metabolic process known as glycolysis. The lactate and hydrogen ions produced in the process are collectively known as lactic acid. While the human body is well-equipped to deal with lactic acid, good nutrition also helps to reduce its impact faster.

Rest/sleep

A few nights of inadequate sleep may not seem like much, but you'd be surprised at how quickly it can derail your diet and training goals. Sleeping well after a workout is critical and can help your body grow stronger, burn fat faster, and make you feel more energized during the day. But to reap these benefits, we need to get consistent sleep every night if possible. If you don't get enough, you may be too tired to exercise during the day and not want to work out.

Chapter 7
Gear Up: Basic Equipment You Need

"Tools evidence the limitations of our bare hands. But they also evidence the creativity of a determined mind."

- Craig D. Lounsbrough

Doing things from home has never been as easy as in 2022. We can work from home, shop from there, study, and meet new people without stepping outside, technically. So, why shouldn't the same apply to exercise and fitness? It's true; not everyone likes gyms. Some are crowded; others are intimidating. The noise is just too much for some of us, and the fees aren't for everybody either. You might be short of time too, and need to stack in a few minutes of S&C.

Fortunately, we can save ourselves time, heartache, and stress from going to the gym every time we need to exercise. We only need a few purchases to create a personalized "gym" in the comfort of our homes. Most, if not all, of the equipment discussed in this chapter is affordable and easily found online. As a result, we can do every workout simply and safely in the confines of your home.

These at-home "gym" equipment will help support your fitness goals, from the simplest to the toughest. Remember, you must stick to what works for you because not every method fits everyone.

Before we discuss this equipment, there's one important tip I must share with you;

Buy something you'll use!

AN ELEGANT SOLUTION

The beauty of this book's design is that it enables you to do these exercises from your home or apartment. It's an elegant solution for those looking for a convenient way to get and stay fit. It requires very little space and is designed for simplicity, safety and results. Outside of getting a personal trainer, this book is one of the most comprehensive workout solutions you'll be able to find anywhere. I still encourage you to read all you can about the subject, whether it's a blog, article, or another book.

The following are the tools/equipment you'll need to accomplish the mission at home.

A Chair

Are you looking for simple ways to fit in a workout? Pull a chair. Yes, some exercises will need us to have a chair; with it, we can target your whole body. The chair will help us burn calories, create a firm midsection, and even build muscles.

Chairs are significant when we have mobility and balance issues. Because the chair provides extra support, we can easily target our lower bodies. And when mentioning a chair, it's not just for working our legs. We can also work our upper body, including arms, chest, and shoulders. Moreover, chairs are the perfect partners for seated stretches. We can hold it for support if we like; we'll be able to do much.

And the best part is that chairs make workouts very convenient. You can grab it, carry it and do a little stretching and simple weight lifting anywhere; living room, kitchen, bedroom, you name it.

Yoga Mat (or carpeted floor)

So yesterday, you were contented doing a few sit-ups or stretches on the linoleum floor, but when you woke up today, you had a kink in your back. What happened? You probably hurt yourself trying to exercise on a hard surface. This is why we need an exercise mat or a carpeted floor at the very least.

A nice comfy yoga mat will provide the necessary solace as you exercise. And who wants to lay down on a dirty floor when they are already sweaty? (And you will sweat). In addition, the extra layer of protection provided by yoga mats will protect your joints from unnecessary injuries and irritations. This is particularly important for people who have sensitive joints.

A mat stabilizes our bodies so we don't slip and fall, especially when doing more complex yoga or stretching. Buy a mat if safety, support, and comfort are a priority for you.

Foam Roller

Have you heard of the SMR (self-myofascial release) technique? I haven't touched on it yet, but SMR is a fancy word used to describe self-massage methods popular in the fitness industry today. Foam rollers are the most common equipment used in SMR.

They are also suitable for floor exercises, especially those that help with lower back pain or sore shoulders by promoting relaxation and increasing blood floor to muscles and other tissues. I love foam rollers for massaging my calf muscles, where I have chronic tightness and muscle soreness.

The process of "foam rolling" targets soft tissue, including fascia and muscles, so we can easily use them to work almost all major muscle groups, including the upper back, hams, calves, and quadriceps. In addition, we can relieve ourselves of soreness and inflammation and increase our joint range of motion by using foam rollers. So add foam rolling to your cool-downs, warm-ups, and even while watching television.

Towel

Towels may sound self-explanatory because they are an obvious part of workout etiquette. But why mention it here?

As you already know, towels act as a barrier and provide a layer of protection between us and the millions of germs we expose ourselves to when working out. They can also keep us cool during exercise and dry our sweating hands, so we don't drop equipment when working out.

Towels may look like random accessories, but when used correctly, towels can help us work our shoulders, arms, lats, and even legs. We can also use them like resistance bands. Simply twist the towel into a rope-like shape, and voila, a resistance band. When rolled up, towels can also provide extra support when doing floor exercises and are helpful in place of cushions such as wedges and bolsters.

Towels can also be improvised and used as sliders so we can glide across the floor easily while working on our balance and core muscles. Towels won't work well as gliders on carpeted floors. Instead, try using them on laminated, vinyl, and hardwood floors. When rolled up, towels also provide extra support when doing challenging yoga poses. Towels are affordable, easily-accessible, multi-functional, and fitness aids.

Light Weights: 1-5 lbs. dumbbells

We can build muscle and improve endurance using lighter weights. We can also buy dumbbells, stability of medicine balls, or bands. Even when the weights are lighter, the benefits are still extensive. Working out with light weights helps define the muscles, giving our joints more functionality. They help us burn calories and provide sustainable workout options that we can maintain for a long time.

Optional (but encouraged): Resistance Bands, Bench, Dowel/Broomstick, and Exercise Ball

Resistant bands are affordable, safe, portable, and easy to use in the comfort of your home. They'll help us build muscle and burn calories. In fact, we can work almost every muscle in our body with a resistance band. The resistance offered by bands differs depending on the thickness. The thicker the band, the more resistance it is likely to offer.

Benches offer the support we need when doing resistance workouts. With them, we can improve the quality and variety of our workouts. It is a versatile home gym equipment that we should all consider.

Exercise balls are great for core muscles and improve balance, flexibility, and coordination. In addition, they help with posture, so we have more stability as we work out.

Clothing

You'll need some loose-fitting, breathable materials and supportive shoes for exercise. Please avoid using socks as they don't have the necessary support and may cause shin splints. Socks also tend to slip on yoga mats.

Look for cotton, bamboo, nylon, and polyester fabrics. Of course, don't be limited to these fabrics, but they offer great comfort and breathability.

Find the clothing that improves your performance. Always try something on to make sure it feels good. If it doesn't make you feel comfortable and confident, try something else that fits well.

Chapter 8
The Exercises: Head to Toe

"Good things come to those who sweat."

- Anonymous

Throughout this book, we've talked comprehensively about all the habits we can adopt into our lives to increase longevity. We've mentioned all the simple tweaks we can make in our movements, diets, and mindset to improve our health. That is the main focus of this book, particularly how strength and conditioning can help us.

FORM AND FUNCTION

It's a great feeling of accomplishment when we can grab a bigger dumbbell, walk or run an extra mile, walk a whole flight of stairs, or add another set of plates to our weights. But, that said, I must tell you that there are some counterproductive ways to exercise, especially when lifting weights. And they can lead to negative results, harm joints, tear muscles, and slow recovery or preventative maintenance processes. So, posture (form) and breathing are critical.

Learning the wrong thing (hopefully through observation) is essential to avoid it. An incorrect posture is not only a setup for inefficiency but can also lead to injuries. We may even find that we exercise the wrong muscles with bad posture. If our exercise mechanics are sound, we'll find that our S&C training is more focused, efficient, and of course, safer.

Some common mistakes people make when exercising include:

Bad neck posture

Many people bend their necks backward when working out. For example, they look up when doing a pushup or a deadlift. Poor neck posture can cause cervical spine injury. The best way to do it would be to "pack" the neck. First, ensure the chin points downward slightly, forming a double chin. Then, work out with the neck in that position.

In most cases, it's safest to keep your eyes forward. This is because your head tends to follow where your eyes go, and your body follows where your head is. Keeping this rule in mind helps 90% of any struggles with posture and form. You'll see this reminder in most of our exercise descriptions.

Pushing overhead with an arched back

It is a common thing; many people bend backward to push overhead. Unfortunately, this is a setup for injury and puts much stress on the spine. To do this right, we must squeeze our core, and glutes and push overhead. This option is safe, allowing us to push more weight by stabilizing our lower back.

Jogging on our heels

Jogging on heels is terrible form. It is the simplest way to rattle the knees, hips, and ankles. Repetitive jogging on heels leads to knee pains, ankle injuries, and shin splints. Not just that, it's inefficient, tiring us sooner than we like. This way, our endurance is not put to full use.

Instead, we should learn to land on the balls of our feet, as you'd do when skipping a rope. The quieter we can run, the better. Our bodies learn to absorb the shock from landing and help injuries caused by overuse.

Proper breathing

There is one main hard and fast rule to remember when exercising and lifting weights. And that is...don't forget to breathe! This rule may sound silly or trite, but many people are just starting will often forget about breathing during a lift or a movement, especially if an exercise requires weights. And sometimes, we become so focused on the movement of the exercise that we forget.

Our minds sometimes think holding our breath will give us greater strength when lifting a heavy weight. However, the opposite is true. For example, when repetitively lifting something overhead, as with the shoulder press, we should inhale as the weight is coming down to the resting position and then exhale when the weight is pushed upward in the lifting position. So never hold your breath in either of those positions.

Of course, there are exceptions to the rule, but if you ever need a "fallback" rule for breathing, always be mindful to breathe comfortably, not too deep, and not too shallow. Just breathe.

This list is by no means exhaustive, but examples should help you start to think about the posture mistakes we could be making while performing various exercises.

MUSCLE GROUPS

What muscle groups are best to work out together and why?

S&C conditioning targets the muscles, which we should do 2-3 times weekly for optimal health. Our muscles need both exercise and rest to function well. For this reason, it's sometimes a good idea to work out specific muscle groups together as we let others rest. When we do this, we give our muscles enough recovery time.

There's also the "whole body" approach, where the 2-3 times you exercise per week involves using exercises that hit all the muscle groups at once. Both systems work, and both have pros and cons.

Why should we exercise specific muscle groups together?

Well, the whole point of strength and condition training is improving the strength of specific muscles through targeted exercise. And to function optimally, many muscles work together. For example, we target chest muscles when doing pushups. However, other muscles like the triceps and shoulders are often involved in the same exercise. When we target only a single muscle, the supportive muscles can suffer neglect. The supporting muscles are used just as much as the "main" muscle. So, when we are trying to strengthen our chest muscles, other muscles are getting some work too.

Our bodies have over 600 muscles. Regarding strength training, most people target six to seven different muscle groups. They are:

- Shoulders
- Back
- Chest
- Arms
- Abs
- Hips
- Legs

We can break down these individual groups to target further (see diagram). These aren't an exhaustive list but include the main muscles (and their abbreviated names) associated with the above groups:

- Shoulders: Trapezius (Traps), Deltoids (Delts)
- Back: Latissimus Dorsi (Lats)
- Chest: Pectorals (Pecs)
- Arms: Biceps (Bis), Triceps (Tris), Forearms
- Abs: Obliques
- Hips: Gluteus (Glutes)
- Legs: Hamstrings, Quadriceps (Quads), Calves

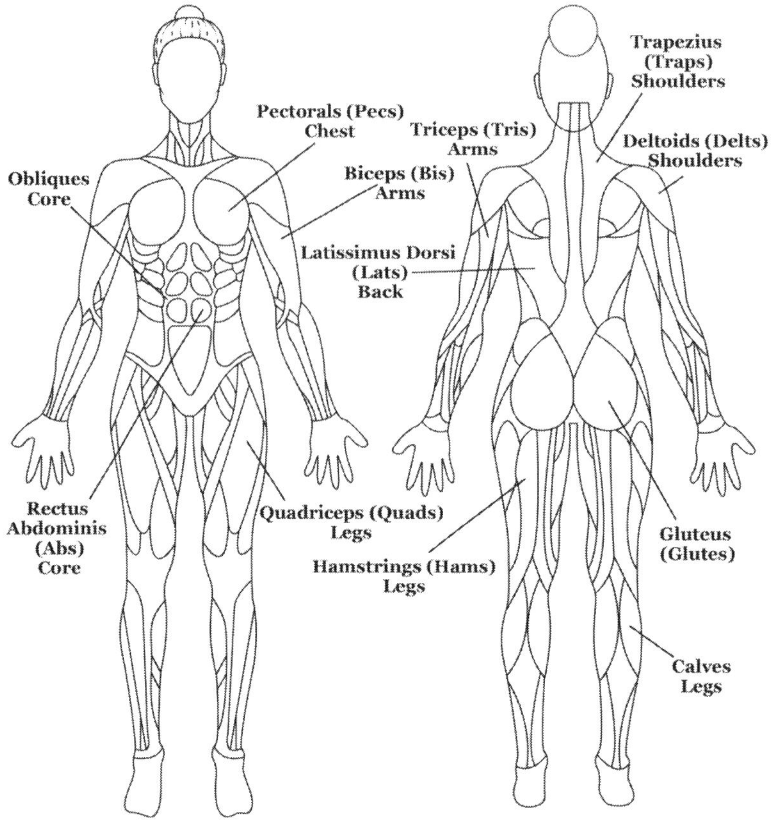

There are many ways to group muscles. For example, some experts will group muscles by their muscle's pull and push functionality. Others look to group them based on their physical location in the body.

Here are some common muscle groupings:

The push muscles are the chest, triceps, and shoulders. More often than not, we exercise these muscles when we push weights away from the body with resistance. Bench press and pushups are good examples of workouts that target push muscles.

The pull muscles, which are the biceps and back, are used in pulling weight/resistance towards the body. Many exercises, including pull-downs, engage the pull muscles.

The hamstrings, legs, glutes (butt), calves, and quadriceps are the leg muscles, which most people give a whole day to exercise. Many workouts engage multiple muscles during a single exercise. An excellent workout should engage all leg muscles.

The abs. Some targeted muscles train the abs, but other exercises train the abs along with other muscles.

In this chapter, the "head to toe" will take us through the exercises based on muscle groups. We will organize these groups into four categories as follows:

- Upper Body: Neck, Shoulders, Upper Back, Chest Arms
- Core, Balance
- Lower Body: Low Back, Hips, Glutes, Quads, Hamstrings, Calves

- Full Body

How much time to put into each workout routine and why?

This question is one of the most commonly asked by people interested in working out. The problem with that question is that there is no simple, straightforward answer. The answer is, it depends! Remember, no single workout is perfect for everybody, but we can at least find common ground regarding the issue of time.

When answering this challenging question, there are a few things we must consider:

Fitness levels

What's your overall fitness level? If you are a beginner, daily spending hours in the gym may come with more significant risks than rewards. You'll burn out, push your body too far too soon, or get injured. Beginners may want to start with shorter workouts, 30 minutes or less. Even if you can only muster 10-15 mins, do it. Any movements are good movements. As our strength grows, we can add more minutes to our workouts.

According to the American Heart Association, the typical adult should perform at least 75-150 minutes of strength training and aerobic activity weekly. The same suggestions recommend at least three 40-minute workout sessions per week. If it's too much, then even 15 minutes will do. It's better to complete even a 10-minute workout than to not do anything. Remember, any movement is good movement.

Type of exercise

How strenuous is the exercise? The more intense a workout is, the lesser time we'll spend on it. So, for example, it's not impossible to maintain a 40-minute brisk walk on the treadmill but good luck maintaining a sprint on the treadmill for that long.

Even if we want to spend more time at the gym, we must think about the workouts carefully. Then, we can go for the shorter, high-intensity workouts on busy days and do low-intensity workouts when we have time.

Rest

If you've been to the gym, you've probably seen some people who look like they are doing nothing other than just standing and idling. However, you may not know that these people are actually resting between sets, and it'd be good for us to do the same.

Some exercises, particularly weightlifting, need rest, recovery, and preparation. While someone may be doing a 30-minute weightlifting session, only 20 minutes involve actual lifting. Add at least 10 minutes to every S&C training session you have. We'll use the extra ten for stretching, recovery, and rest.

Commitments

The most important question is, how much do we prioritize exercise, and how much time are we willing to put in? Our health should come first, and we should invest in it. I know family and career are important, and we may find ourselves cutting short an exercise routine to attend to other matters. That's okay.

As we know, even 10 minutes of workout is better than no workout. So be proud of whatever you have time for, no matter how the workout is.

What is progressive overload?

Our bodies constantly adapt to our exercise routine, no matter what. Therefore, to be effective, we must modify our workouts over time as our bodies get used to the older challenges.

Progressive overload is the gradual increase in the number of repetitions, frequency, and weights in our S&C training or any other exercise. By doing this, our bodies slowly adapt to the new challenges and become stronger over time.

Progressive overload is the best way to keep your body from plateauing. Plateauing is where our bodies get used to the workout we've been doing over time, so our bodies don't get as many benefits from that exercise as they used to. Progressive overload counters this, so we become stronger and fitter as you continue working out.

Plateauing is good because it shows that you have achieved a particular fitness milestone, but we must shake things up a little when it happens. For example, you can increase the size of your weights and frequency of your workouts as soon as you notice that your body no longer benefits from the regular exercises you've been doing. You can also change to a different exercise that focuses on the muscle group(s) you're trying to develop.

Disclaimer

Your health comes first. To do any of the workouts mentioned in this book, you should be physically healthy with no medical complications or impairments that might impede your workout plans. I cannot give medical advice. My goal is to offer you the best exercises, workout programs, nutritional information, and how to best achieve the goals you set for yourself. My goal is not to advise you about your personal physical health or ability, to do any of the workouts mentioned, or to give you detailed nutritional plans for your body in this book. So please consult your doctor before exercising or starting a training program.

THE EXERCISES

As mentioned in Chapter 6, breathing and posture are critical to the success of our workouts. So, it will benefit us to revisit them once more in the context of the specific exercises ahead.

Your form should match the illustrations as best as possible, knowing that these will always be a work in progress. Movement should be fluid and steady with no erratic or jerky motions. Please note that many of these exercises can be done seated or standing. Do not hold your breath. Breathing should be slow, steady, and relaxed throughout the exercises.

Lastly, before diving in, some of these exercises will feel foreign until you've worked on them for a bit. So please do not become discouraged if you can't get them immediately. Also, it is always a good practice to have a chair handy for any additional balance that might be needed, especially early on in the learning process.

Strength Exercises

- Upper Body
- Core
- Lower Body
- Full Body

The exercises in this section will help increase your strength in specific areas. These are called strength exercises, and there are hundreds more than you see here. However, I've cherry-picked these exclusively for this book. Our stretching and warm-up exercises will directly follow the strength exercises from head to toe.

Each of the following exercises has many physical benefits, from strengthening and toning muscles to stress relief. And each one of them often benefits multiple muscle groups and joints.

Each exercise contains illustrations showing the mechanics of each movement. In addition, the text will outline the "body part" they affect, the "benefit" of the exercise, and a description of "how to" perform it. You will also see the recommended number of repetitions (reps) if you want to do these separately from a workout. In the workout chapter (Ch 9), these numbers of reps may change slightly since we're doing several exercises together within the workouts.

Finally, I encourage you to try all these exercises to see which ones benefit you the most. Then, in addition to the individual workouts in Chapter 9, you can start crafting your own workouts based on your needs and goals. Think of the following exercises as items on a menu that you can select for your "workout meal," similar to a "pick 3" or an ala carte approach to dining.

Upper Body Strength Exercises

Exercise: Neck Side Press

Body Part: Neck

Benefit: Helps posture, head movement, and upper spine strength.

How To: While keeping your eyes looking forward and shoulders square, put your palm on one side of your head and resist by pushing your head into your hand. Keep your head as still as possible. Do both sides for 10-15 seconds each.

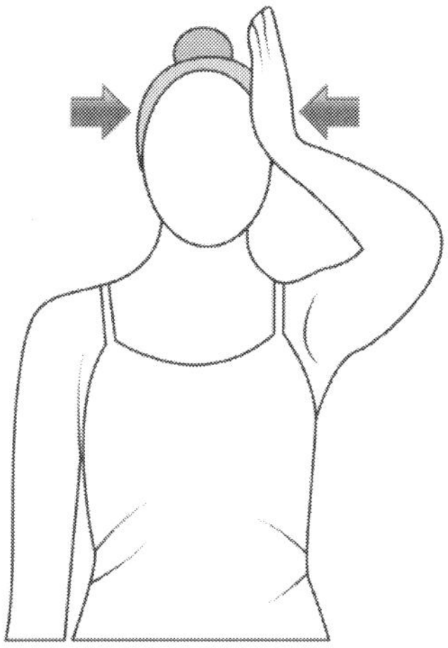

Exercise: Neck Front and Back Press

Body Part: Neck

Benefit: Helps posture, head movement, and upper spine strength.

How To: While keeping your shoulders square and back straight, place the palm of your hand on your forehead and push to create resistance. Do this for 10 seconds. Next, put your hand on the back of your head and push back into your hand. Keep your back and neck straight. Do this for 10 seconds.

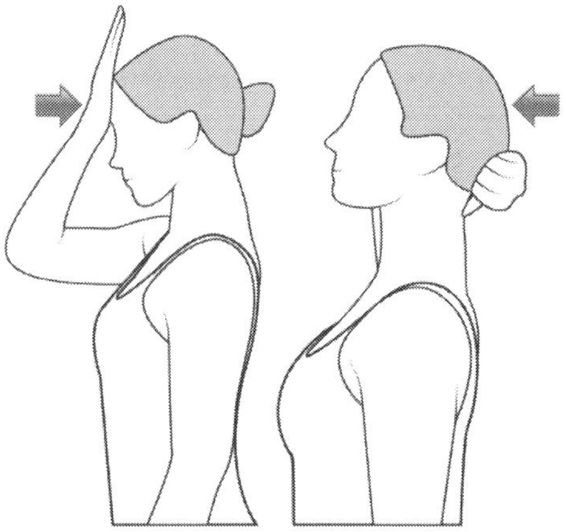

Exercise: Shoulder Squeezes

Body Part: Neck, Shoulders

Benefit: Helps posture, shoulder, and mid-back strength

How To: Stand straight, with feet shoulder-width apart. Draw your shoulders back while squeezing your shoulder blades together. Hold while squeezing for 10 seconds, then release back to the relaxed position. Do this 10-12 times.

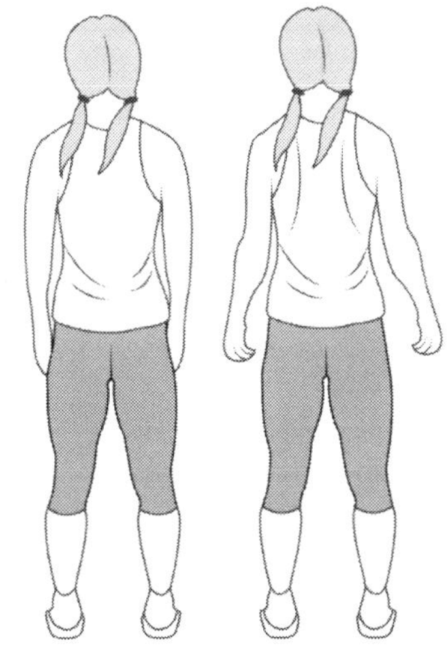

Exercise: Arm Circles (various sizes)

Body Part: Shoulders

Benefit: Increases toning in the shoulders and back, keeps shoulder joints limber.

How To: Standing with your feet shoulder-width apart, hold your arms straight out, and then rotate them while making medium-sized circles. Do 15 forward circles, then 15 backward. You can also change the size of your circles from large or small.

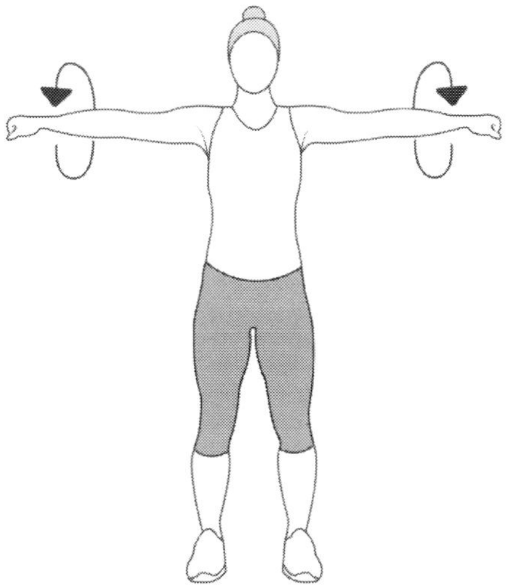

Exercise: Arm Swings

Body Part: Shoulders, Chest, Upper Back

Benefit: Increases strength and flexibility in the shoulders and chest and warms up multiple upper body parts.

How To: While standing straight with feet slightly shoulder width apart, extend your arms parallel to the floor. Next, bring your arms across your front like scissors and bring them back to the original position. Do 15-20 reps changing the arm that's on top each time.

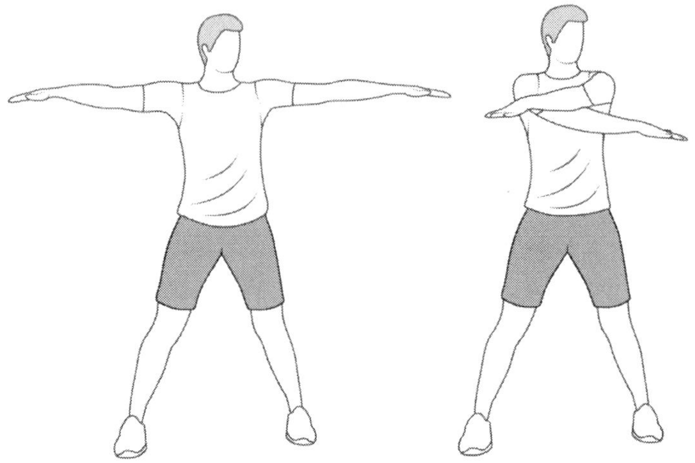

Exercise: Car Drivers

Body Part: Shoulders, Upper Back, Neck

Benefit: Increases shoulder, upper back, and lower neck strength and toning.

How To: This can be done with a book or any flat object with some weight. Start with approx.1-2 pounds. With feet shoulder-width apart, head forward, and arms parallel to the ground, place your hands at 3 and 9 o'clock. Move the object away from you with arms fully extended. Rotate the object to the right to about 12 o'clock and then back to the left, again at 12 o'clock. Do this 8-12 times.

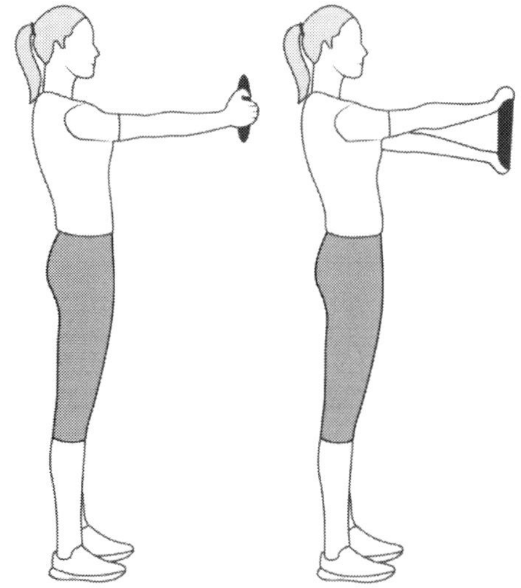

Exercise: Shoulder Rolls (forward and backward)

Body Part: Shoulders

Benefits: Increases rotator cuff and upper spine flexibility and helps relieve shoulder stress and pain.

How To: Sitting straight up with hands at your sides, roll your shoulders forward for one full circular rotation and then go backward for another. You can also do multiple rotations in one direction, then reverse it. 15-20 reps are the goal here.

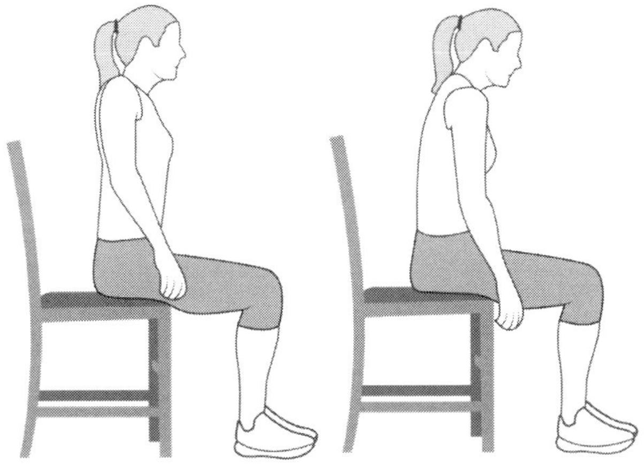

Exercise: Front Shoulder Raises

Body Part: Shoulders, Neck

Benefits: Strengthens and tones shoulders and upper back.

How To: Using light dumbbells, water bottles, or nothing at all, stand straight up with your shoulders slightly back and a slight arch in your back. Slowly raise one arm just past parallel to the ground and then back down. Alternate with the other arm using the same motion. Do this 12-15 times each arm. Be careful not to rock or use your body weight to force the weight up, using only your shoulders to bring up the weight.

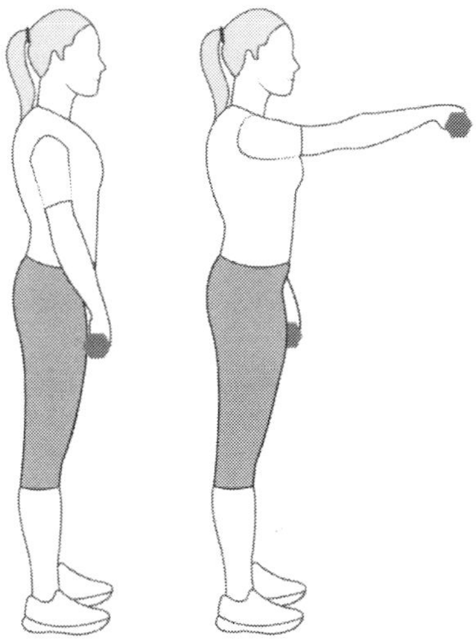

Exercise: Side Shoulder Raises

Body Part: Shoulders, Neck

Benefits: Strengthens and tones shoulders and upper back, and helps with balance.

How To: Similar to Front Shoulder Raises, you can use a light weight or no weight. The motion is more important than how much you lift. With your arms at your sides, slowly lift your hands/weights to just past parallel to the ground. Be sure to breathe in when lifting up and out when coming down. 12-15 times is a good goal. Again, do not rock your body.

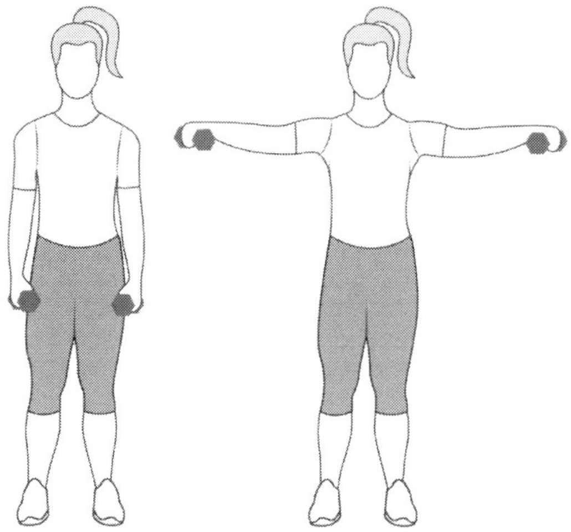

Exercise: Shoulder Shrugs

Body Part: Shoulders, Neck

Benefits: Strengthens shoulders, trapezius muscle (neck), and upper back, and helps with neck strain.

How To: Holding your hands at your sides (with small weights like dumbbells or water bottles), keep your head still and forward, and slowly shrug your shoulders towards your ears. Maintain the shrug for 3-5 seconds, then come back down. Do this 12-15 times. This exercise is good together with arm circles.

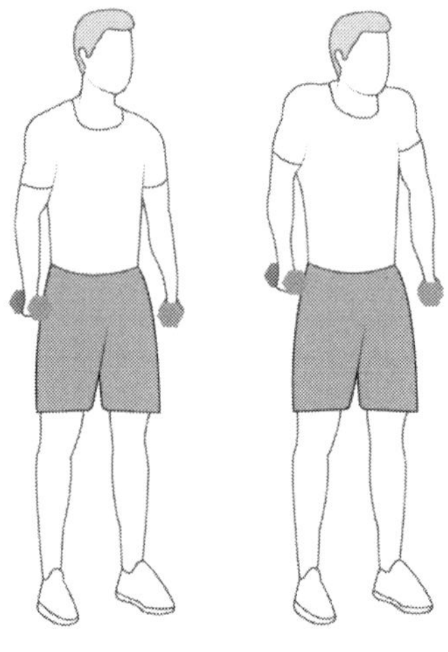

Exercise: Overhead Shoulder Press

Body Part: Shoulders, Upper Back

Benefits: Strengthens and tones shoulders, upper back, and a small amount of the arms and chest.

How To: With your head forward and arms holding small weights or nothing (making a fist), start with elbows bent just past 90 degrees and palms facing inward. Slowly press the weight upward until your arms are fully extended, and then slowly come back down and repeat. Try to keep your back from arching too much, as the lift should come from your shoulders. Aim for 12-15 reps. You can also do this same exercise with palms facing outward for variety.

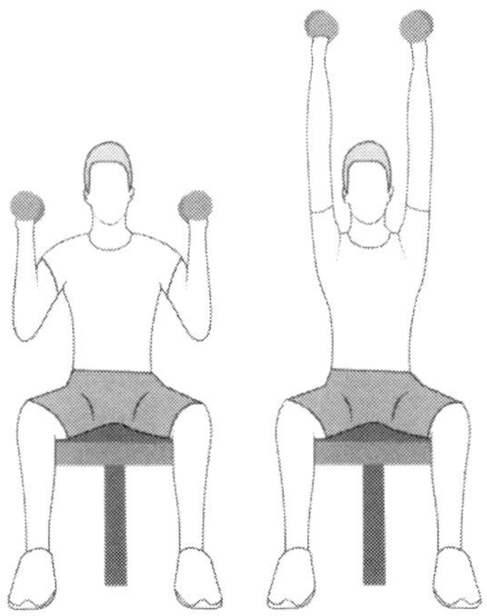

Exercise: Wall Angels

Body Part: Shoulders, Upper Back

Benefit: Strengthens upper back, spine, and shoulders and helps with posture.

How To: With your back against a wall, put your hands up and bend your arms to 90 degrees. Keeping your feet shoulder-width apart, slowly reach toward the ceiling keeping your arms and shoulder blades flat against the wall. Come back down in the same slow motion making sure your arms and blades stay against the wall. This exercise is good for practicing breathing and helping to relieve stress. Do this 10-12 times.

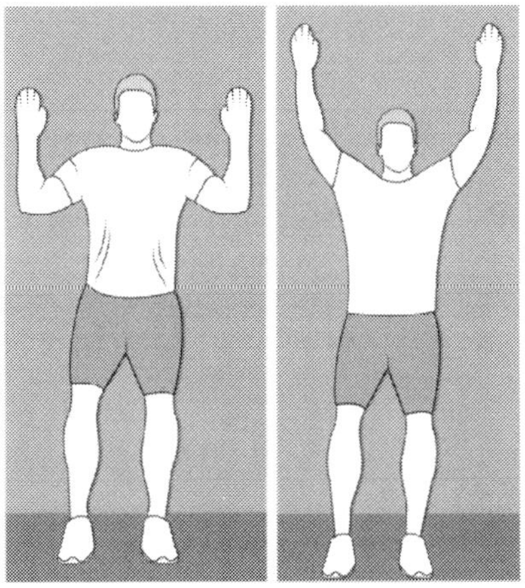

Exercise: Bent Over Rows

Body Part: Upper Back (Lats), Shoulders, Arms

Benefit: Strengthens and tones upper back and shoulders and improves spinal stability.

How To: Using a chair, place one hand on its top and hold a small (or no) weight. Bend the knees and hips to about 45 degrees. Pull the weight up slowly until it reaches your stomach, bringing it back in the same fashion. The key is ensuring your back stays straight or slightly arched but not hunched over. Do these 10-12 times per arm.

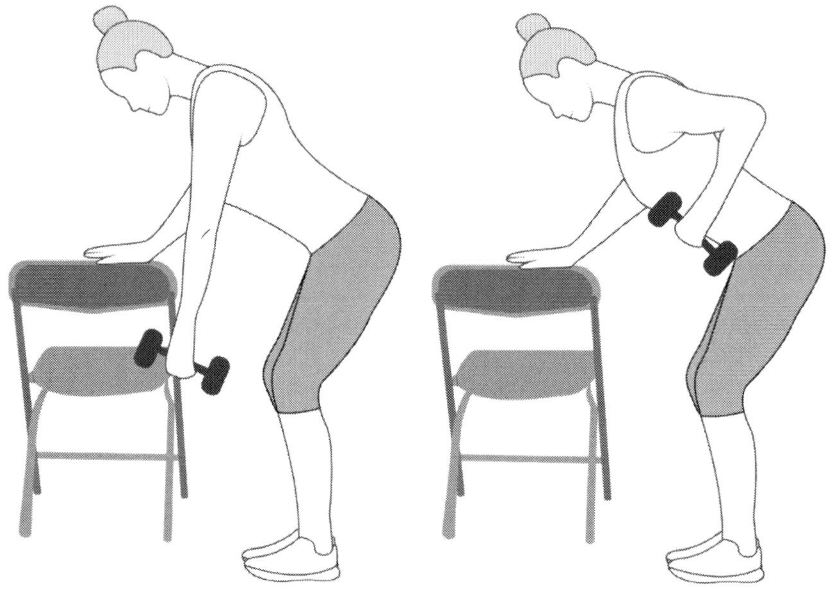

Exercise: Jack Knives

Body Part: Upper Back (Lats), Shoulders, Hips

Benefit: Strengthens shoulders, neck, and upper back and improves spinal and hip stability.

How To: Standing with your feet slightly less than shoulder-width apart, bend at the hips to about 30-40 degrees. Place your arms out and align them with your ears. Slowly pull your elbows down and bring your arms fully extended and then gently straight back. Do this slowly 12-15 times.

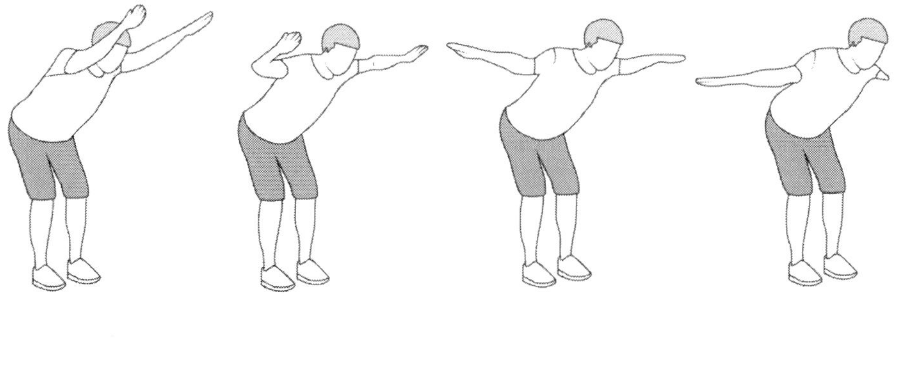

Exercise: Upright Rows

Body Part: Upper Back, Shoulders

Benefit: Strengthen upper back and shoulders and helps with pulling.

How To: Standing with your feet shoulder-width apart, keep eyes forward and arms resting on your thighs, with or without light dumbbells. Holding your weights/hands close to your body, slowly bring your elbows up to where they're pointing straight out from your body, even with your shoulders. You should feel your shoulder blades come together. Pause briefly and come back down slowly to the original position. Do this 10-15 times.

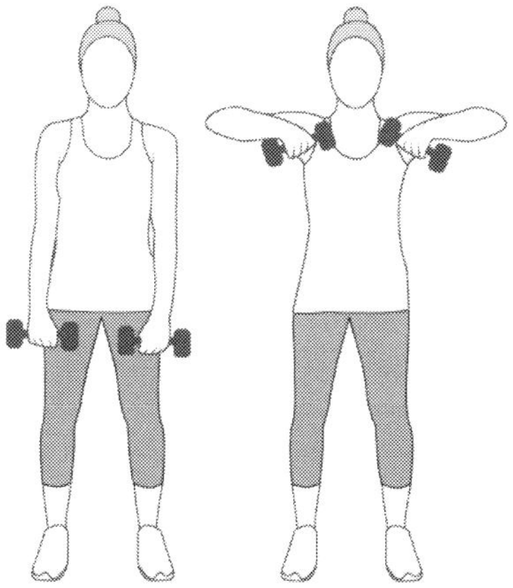

Exercise: Seated Chest Isometrics (Prayer)

Body Part: Chest, Shoulders, Upper Back, Spine

Benefit: Tones chest and shoulders and helps breathing and posture

How To: In a seated position, place your hands in front of you (chest level) in a prayer-like fashion. Gradually push your hands together and when you feel the tension in your chest, breathe deeply and slowly bring your hands up until they are even with your face. Keep pushing your palms together, and slowly exhale, bringing them back down to chest level. Release the tension briefly and then repeat 15 times.

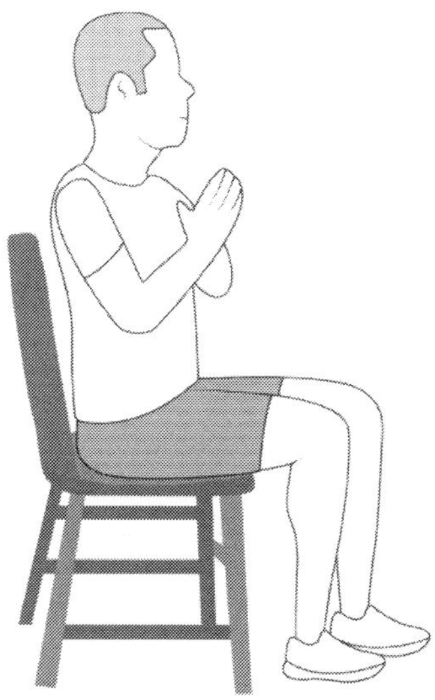

Exercise: Seated Chest Squeeze

Body Part: Chest, Shoulders, Upper Back, Spine

Benefit: Strengthens shoulders, chest, back, helps posture

How To: While seated, place your arms at a 90-degree angle in front of you. Hands can be open or closed. Slowly bring your elbows together, pause, and then bring your arms slowly upward until your elbows are about eye level. Slowly bring your elbows back down and open your arms to the original position. Repeat this 12-15 times.

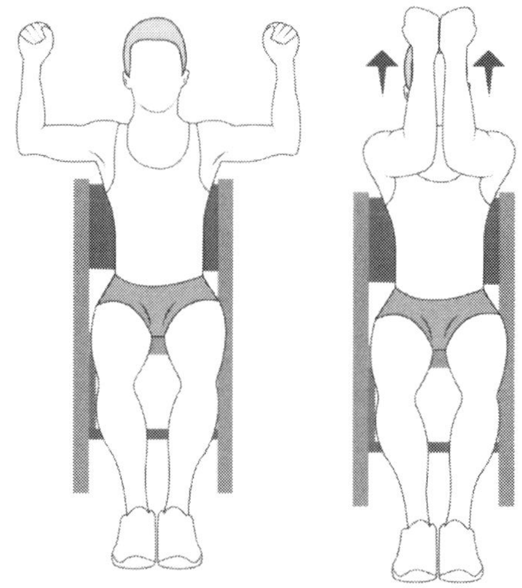

Exercise: Chest Openers

Body Part: Chest, Upper Back, Shoulders, Spine

Benefit: Tones and strengthens the chest, shoulders, and back and helps with posture and breathing/relaxing.

How To: Standing with your arms closed, palms together, and parallel to the ground, keep your eyes forward. Take a deep breath and open your arms just past your body while pushing your chest slightly. You should feel your chest open up. Pause here, exhale and take another deep breath, then return to the original position. Do this 12-15 times.

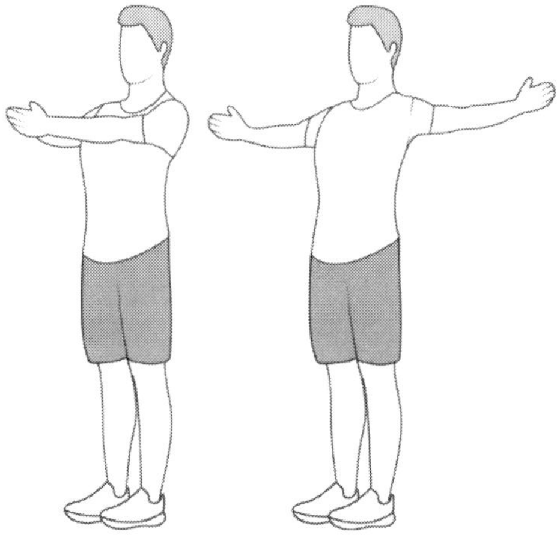

Exercise: Wall PushUps

Body Part: Chest, Arms, Shoulders, Upper Back, Wrists

Benefit: Helps strengthen the pushing muscles and can help with balance. Easier to do than floor pushups.

How To: With your feet shoulder-width apart, roughly 2-3 feet away from the wall, slowly place your hands on the wall just below the shoulders. Keeping your arms slightly bent, back straight, and eyes looking ahead at the wall, slowly bend your elbows until your nose barely touches the wall. Then, slowly push back up to your original position. Do this 12-15 times. If you want to change it up, try varying the width of your hands.

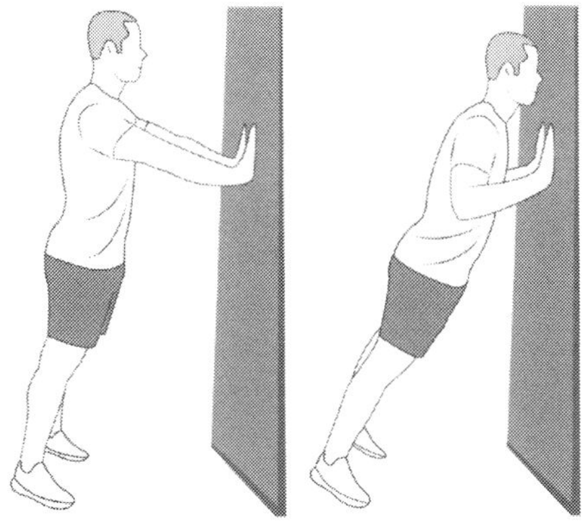

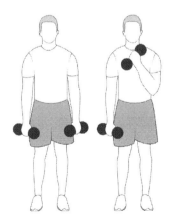

Exercise: Cross Chest Curls

Body Part: Arms (biceps), Chest, Upper Back, Wrist

Benefit: Helps with pulling, grip strength for things like hugging and groceries, and strengthens/tones the beach muscles.

How To: Stand with feet shoulder-width apart and hold a light dumbbell (or no weight) at your sides. Slowly curl your arm up and ever so slightly across your chest towards the opposite shoulder. Once up, slowly bring your arm back down and repeat with the opposite arm. Be careful not to swing your body to bring up the weight and use only your arms and chest. Do this 12-15 times per arm.

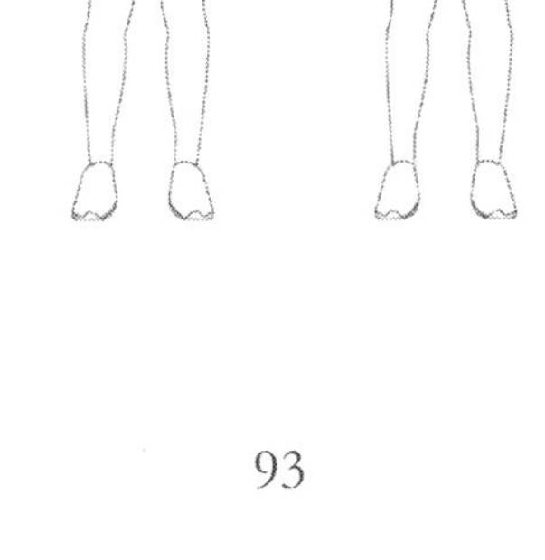

Exercise: Wrist Curl Flexions (palm up)

Body Part: Wrists, Forearms

Benefit: Combats carpal tunnel, improves grip strength

How To: In a seated position, take a light dumbbell in one hand and rest your arm on your thigh and wrist just past your knee, palm facing up. Slowly bend your wrist past your knee towards the floor and then curl the weight up as far as possible, keeping your arm flush with your thigh. Repeat this 12-15 times.

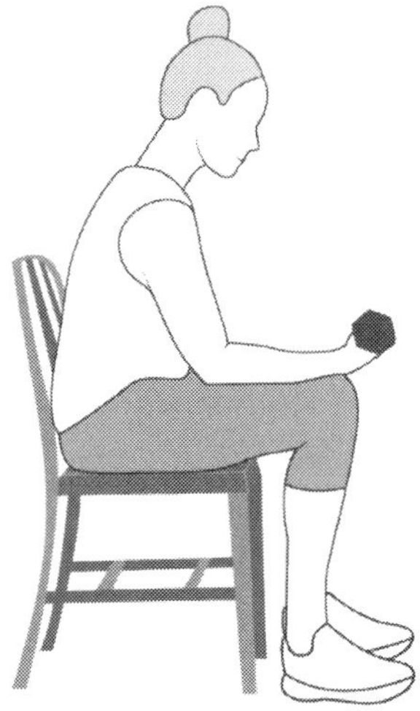

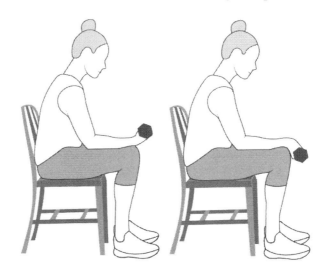

Exercise: Wrist Curl Extensions (palm down)

Body Part: Wrists, Forearms

Benefit: Combats carpal tunnel, improves grip strength

How To: In a seated position, take a light dumbbell in one hand and rest your arm on your thigh and wrist just past your knee, palm facing down. Slowly bend your wrist past your knee towards the floor and then curl the weight up as far as possible, keeping your arm flush with your thigh. Repeat this 12-15 times.

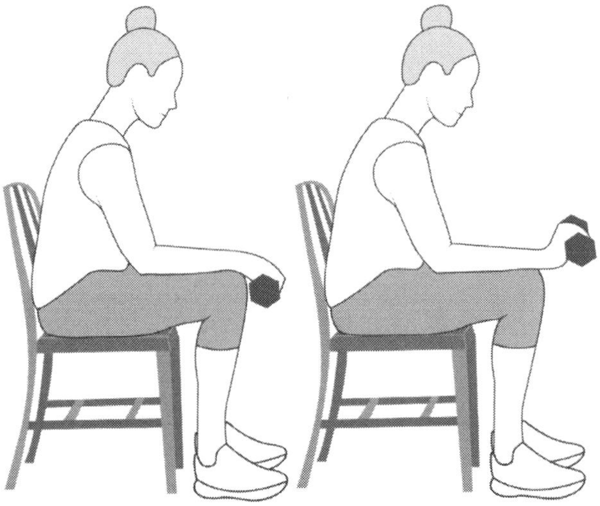

Exercise: Standing Bicep Curls

Body Part: Arms, Shoulder, Upper Back, Wrist

Benefit: Helps with pulling movements and grip strength for things like picking up groceries.

How To: Standing with knees bent slightly, eyes looking forward. With a light dumbbell in each arm, in front of your thighs, bring one arm up slowly towards your shoulder in a curl-like motion. Keep your elbows close to your body. Briefly stop at the top, then slowly return to the original position. Do the same with the other arm, careful not to rock back and forth. Do this 12-15 times per arm.

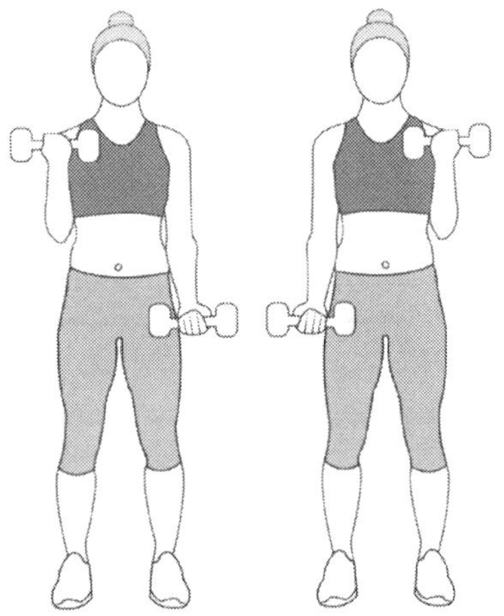

Exercise: Hammer Curls

Body Part: Arms, Shoulders, Upper Back, Wrist

Benefit: Helps with pulling movements and grip strength

How To: This exercise is similar to standing bicep curls, except the hands are turned inward, which works the arms slightly differently. With feet hip-width apart, with a light dumbbell in each arm, rest the weights on your mid-thighs. Slowly lift the dumbbells together until they almost touch your chest. Do this 12-15 times.

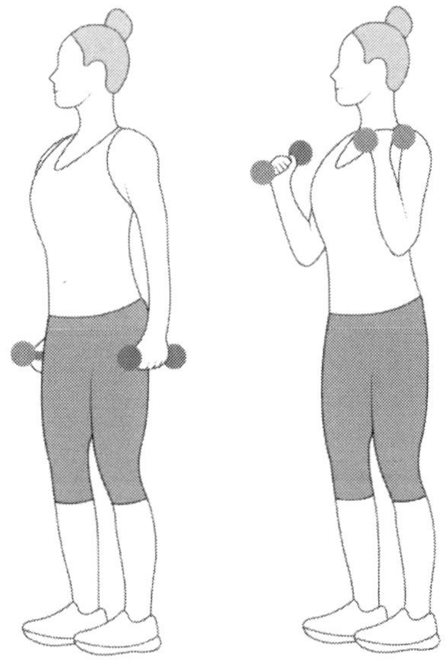

Exercise: Seated Dips

Body Part: Arms (triceps), Chest, Shoulders, Elbows

Benefit: Helps with pushing movements like getting out of a chair, shoulder and elbow joints, and balance.

How To: While sitting, place your hands behind you onto the arms of the chair and scoot to the middle/end of the seat. When ready, slowly push up until your arms are fully extended. Then, slowly return all the way down to the seated position. Do this 12-15 times.

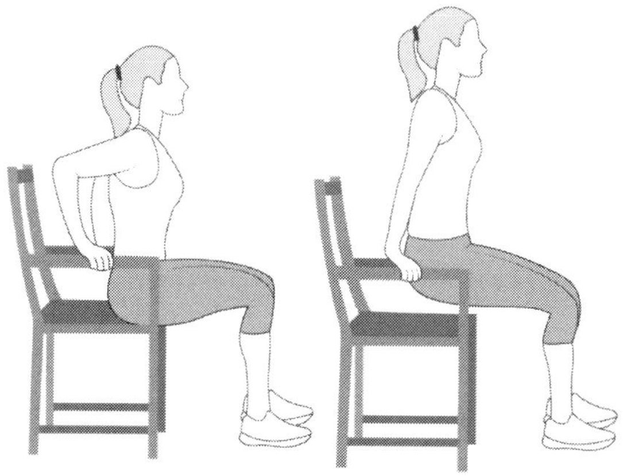

Exercise: Tricep Extensions

Body Part: Arms, Chest, Upper Back, Shoulders, Elbows

Benefit: Helps with pushing movements like lifting things overhead and strengthens shoulder and elbow joints.

How To: Using a light dumbbell, position your hands under the weight and push it overhead with arms extended. Place your feet shoulder-width apart and slowly lower your arms (and weight) down behind your head until your arms are parallel to the floor. You should feel the back of your arms stretch. Slowly push up until you're back up with arms extended. Do this 12-15 times.

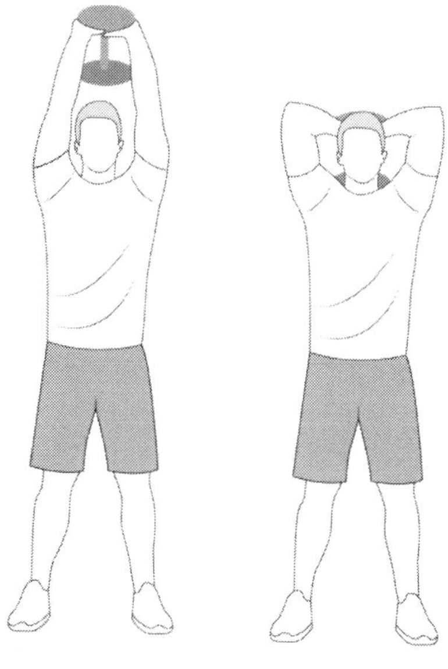

Exercise: Tricep Kickbacks

Body Part: Arms, Upper Back

Benefit: Helps with pushing movements, strengthens and tones the tricep muscles.

How To: Take a light dumbbell in each hand and stand with feet about shoulder width apart. Bend at your waist to about a 45-degree angle. Bring the weights close to your body, bending at the elbows at another 45-degree angle. While keeping your elbows still, slowly take your hands (and weights) back behind you until your arms are fully extended. Make sure to stay in your original bent-over position. Then, slowly bring your weights back to the original spot. Do this 12-15 times.

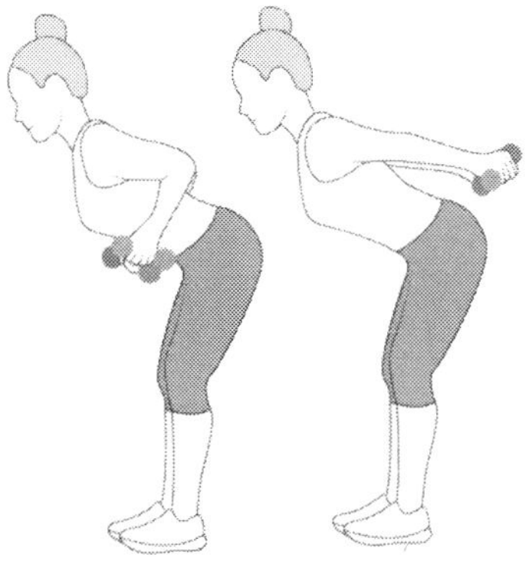

Core Strength Exercises

Exercise: Balance Walking

Body Part: Core, Abs, Hips, Shoulders, Legs

Benefit: Increases balance, awareness, ankle stabilization

How To: With eyes forward and feet shoulder-width apart, bring your arms up, so they are parallel to the floor. Slowly lift up one leg, pointing your knee outward, and hold for 1-2 seconds. Next, slowly put your raised foot forward and down, walking exaggeratedly. The key is to hold your knee up for 1-2 seconds. Repeat this walking motion with the other foot. Do this for 30-60 seconds.

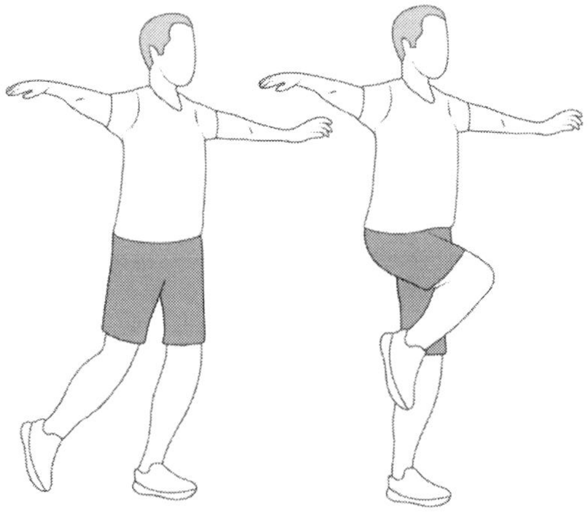

Exercise: The Flamingo

Body Part: Core, Abs, Hips, Legs

Benefit: Increases balance, works hip joints

How To: Standing upright with the back of a chair, place your hands on the top of the chair to stabilize yourself. Next, slowly raise one foot with your knee pointing at the back of the chair. Hold this position for 5-10 seconds. Then, return your foot to the floor slowly and repeat the motion with the other leg. Do this 12-15 times.

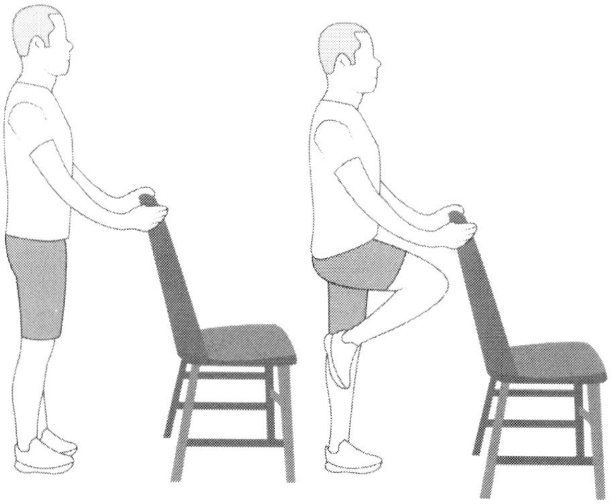

Exercise: Lateral Stepping

Body Part: Core: Hips, Legs

Benefit: Coordination is small spaces, balance

How To: Standing straight with eyes forward and feet close together, grasp the top of a chair's back with one hand. Slowly step to the side opposite of the chair, then slowly step back to the original position. Repeat this ten times, rotate around and do the other leg 10 times.

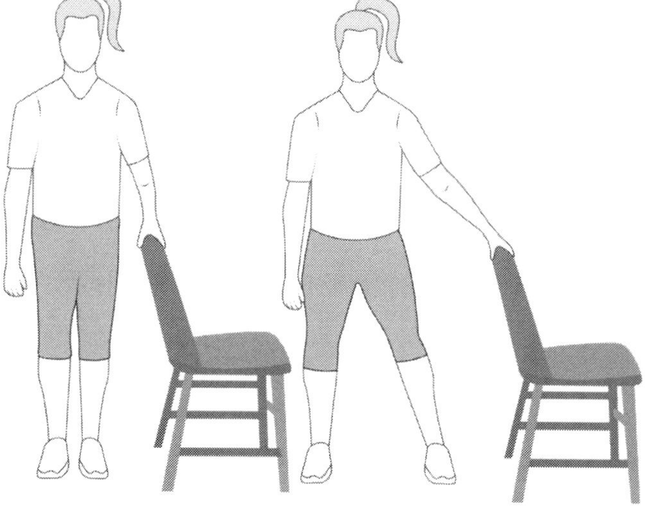

Exercise: Clock Reaches

Body Part: Core, Shoulders, Hips, Legs

Benefit: General balance, coordination, and fixed standing

How To: Standing straight with eyes forward and feet close together, grasp the top of a chair's back with one hand. Imagine you have a "clock's hands," and noon is directly in front of you and 6 o'clock is directly behind you. Slowly raise your outer knee, and slowly raise your hand to the 3 o'clock position (to the side). Next, move your hand slowly to noon and then back to 3. Repeat this motion 5 times, then switch arms and legs.

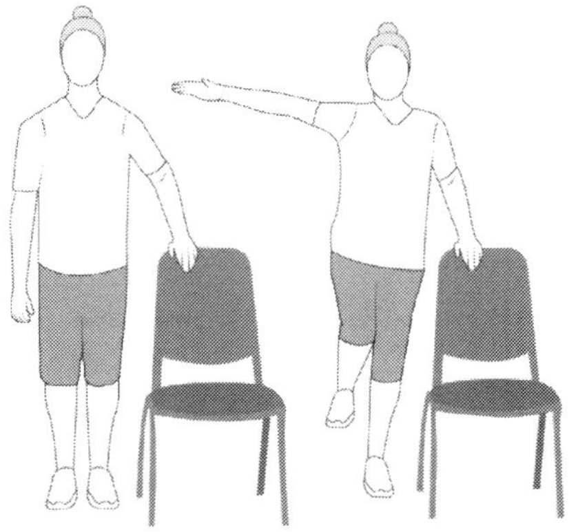

Exercise: The Tightrope

Body Part: Core, Abs, Hips, Legs

Benefit: Improves balance and coordination

How To: Standing straight with one foot in front of the other, place your hands on your hips or out to the side. Slowly put one foot directly in front of the other, with your heel just before your toes. Continue this motion as if walking straight on a tightrope. It may help to use a 6-foot piece of string or yarn as a marker to walk. Do this for 1-2 minutes.

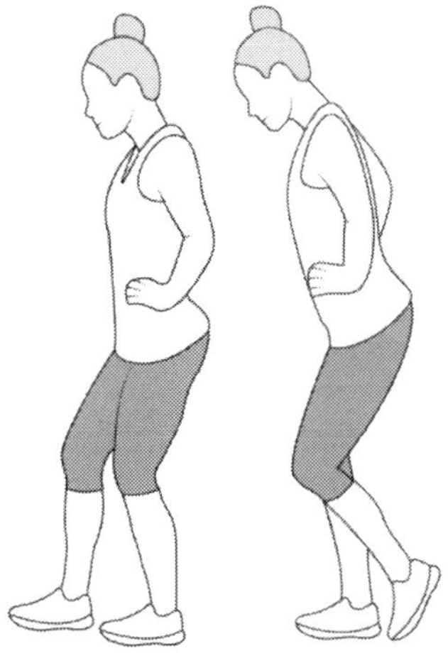

Exercise: Torso Turns

Body Part: Core, Abs, Hips, Low Back, Spine

Benefit: Strengthens and tones core muscles

How To: Looking straight ahead with feet shoulder-width apart, put your palms together and raise them directly in front of you. Keeping your arms parallel to the floor, slowly turn your torso to the left, and hold for 1 second. Slowly rotate back to the right, stopping in the middle at the original spot, then rotate to the right and hold for 1 second. Repeat this full rotation 5 times.

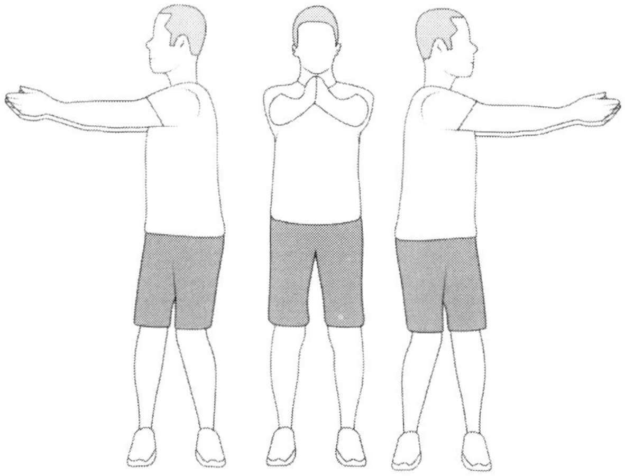

Exercise: Abdominal Bridges

Body Part: Core, Abs, low back, pelvis

Benefit: Strengthens core muscles and lower back

How To: Lying on the floor, rest on your elbows with your hands below your face and pelvis down. Slowly raise your hips, keeping your knees on the floor. Hold in the up position for 1-2 seconds, tighten your abs, then slowly come back down to the floor. Do this 10-12 times.

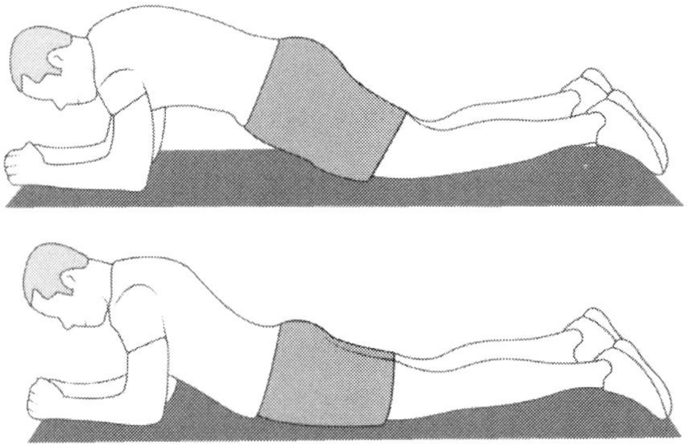

Exercise: Glute Bridges

Body Part: Core, Abs, Glutes,

Benefit: Strengthens core, lower back, and butt

How To: Lying on your back, bend your knees and keep your heels under your knees, and arms at your side. Slowly raise your pelvis until your thighs align with your upper body. On the way up, squeeze your glutes (butt) and abs. Hold at the top for 5-10 seconds. Then, slowly return to the original position. Do this 10 times.

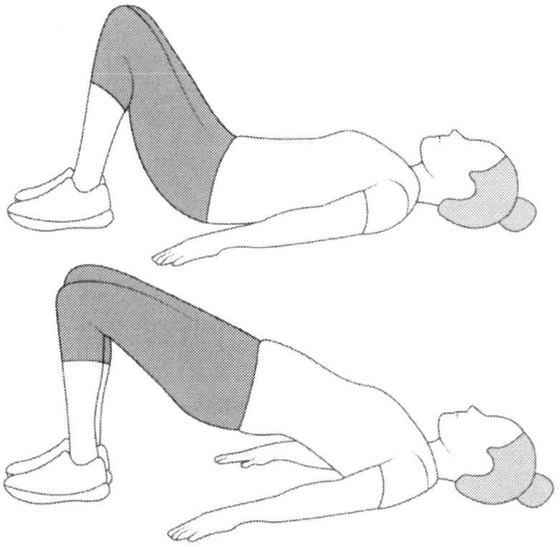

Exercise: Knee to Chest (seated)

Body Part: Core, Abs, Hips, Glutes

Benefit: Helps flexibility in hips and glutes and strengthens core.

How To: Sitting on a chair with your back straight and looking forward, grab one leg with two hands at the back of your thigh, close to your knee. Using your hands as a guide, slowly bring your leg to your chest and try to touch your chest with it. Hold the top position for 4-5 seconds, then slowly come back down. Do this 10 times, then do the other leg 10 times.

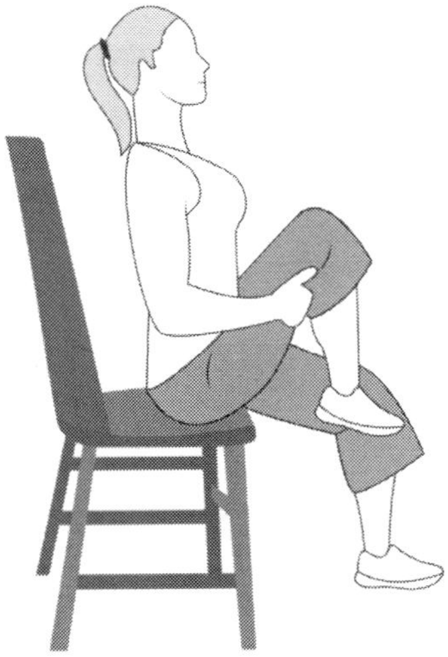

Exercise: Knees to Chest (floor)

Body Part: Core, Abs, Hips, Legs

Benefit:

How To: Lying on your back with your arms at your sides with your knees together, slowly bring your knees to your chest as close as possible. Hold this position for 5-10 seconds, then slowly come back down and do it again 10-12 times. Try not to, but if needed, use your hands to hold your knees up while counting.

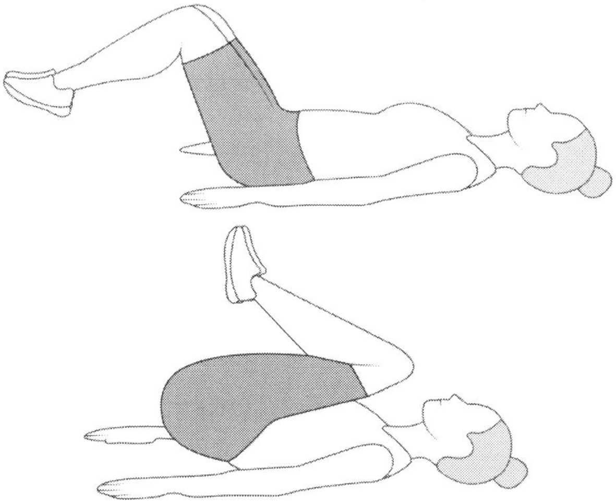

Exercise: Pelvic Tilts

Body Part: Core, Abs, Glutes

Benefit: Strengthens abs, glutes, and pelvis and improves posture

How To: Lying flat on the floor, keep your knees bent, feet and hands flat, and arms at your sides. Slowly arch your back and tilt your hips slightly off the floor. Hold this position for 1-2 seconds and then slowly return to the original spot, with hips flat on the floor. Do this 10 times.

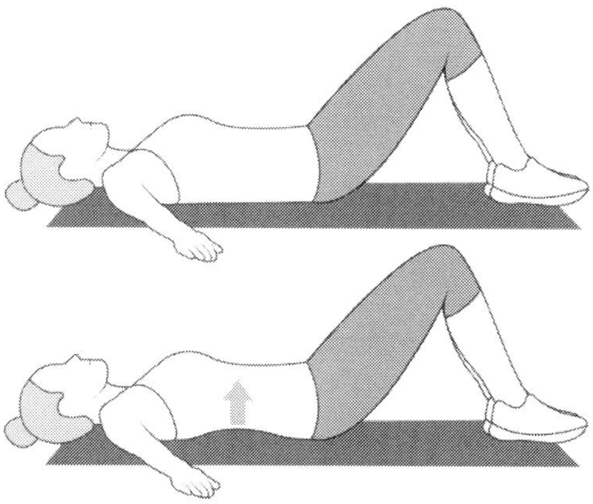

Exercise: Bent Leg Toe Taps

Body Part: Core, Abs, Legs

Benefit: Strengthens and tones core muscles

How To: Lying on your back with arms close to your sides and knees bent, slowly raise both your legs making a 90-degree bend. Keeping one knee still, slowly lower your opposite leg until your toe barely taps the floor. Slowly bring your leg back to the up position and make this same motion with the other leg. Do this 10-12 times each leg.

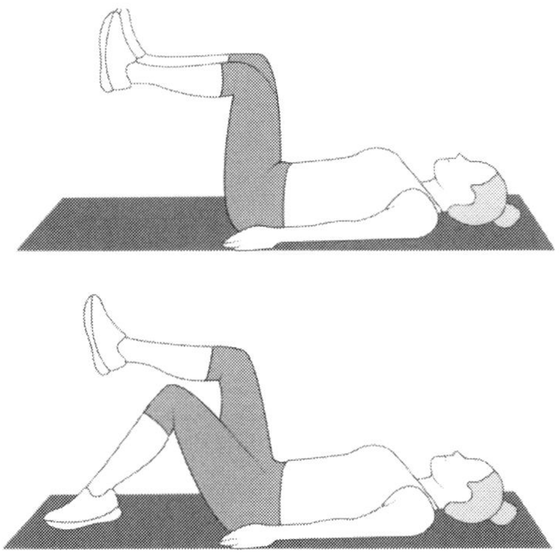

Exercise: Dead Bugs

Body Part: Core, Abs, Shoulders

Benefit: Strengthens and tones core muscles, helps with general coordination

How To: Lying on your back, put your arms straight into the air and raise your legs, so your knees are bent at 90 degrees. Slowly lower one leg so it's straight and just above the floor while lowering the opposite side arm to just above the floor. Slowly alternate the opposite leg and arm to the same positions. Do this 10-15 times.

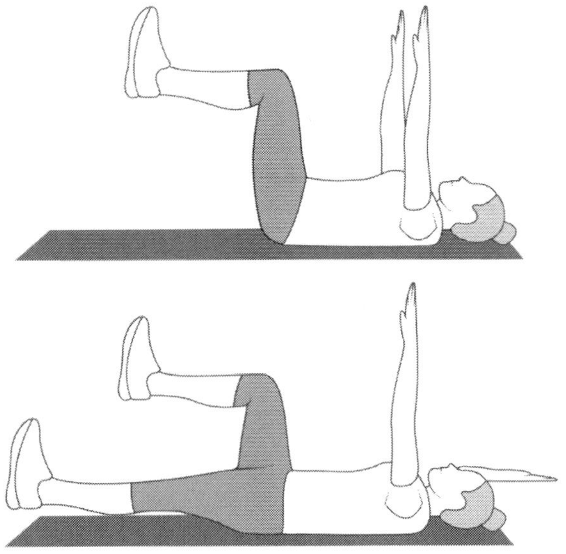

Exercise: The Superman

Body Part: Core, Abs, Back, Legs, Glutes

Benefit: Improves spine stability, tones glutes, helps with posture and reduces low back pain.

How To: Lie with your stomach flat on the floor, with arms out straight and forward, and both legs extended backward. Slowly elevate one arm off the floor while elevating the opposite leg. Then, slowly return them to the floor while elevating the other arm and leg at the same time. Do this 10-15 times.

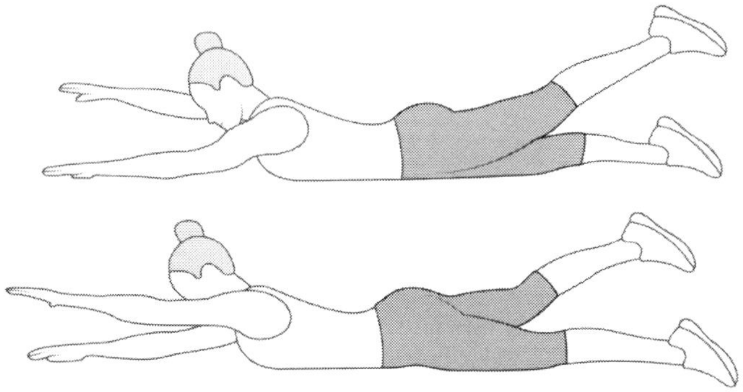

Lower Body Strength Exercises

Exercise: Hands to Knees

Body Part: Lower Back

Benefit: Helps posture, low back pain, strengthens hamstrings

How To: Standing straight up with feet shoulder-width apart, place your palms on the top of your thighs. Slowly bend down from the hips, keeping your knees straight and hands on your thighs until you reach your knees. Keep your back straight. Hold for 1-2 seconds, then slowly return to the original position. Do this 10 times.

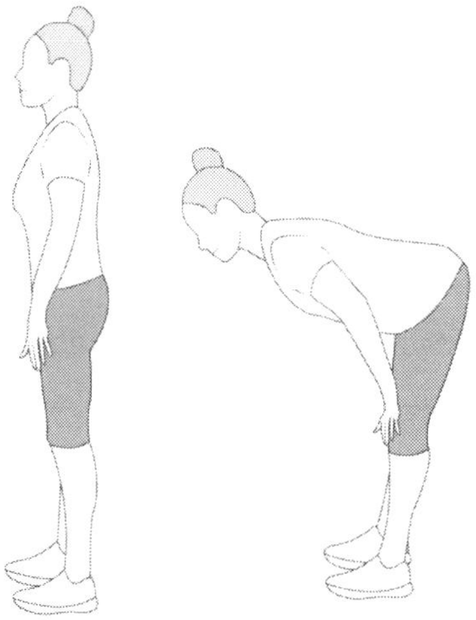

Exercise: The Cobra

Body Part: Lower Back, Abs, Spine

Benefit: Strengthens lower back and spine

How To: Lying prone on the floor, place your hands at your sides by your chest. Very slowly push up while keeping your legs and hips flat. Once your arms are fully extended for 2-3 seconds, you slowly come back down. If your lower back feels too tight after the first rep, go up halfway. Do this 10 times.

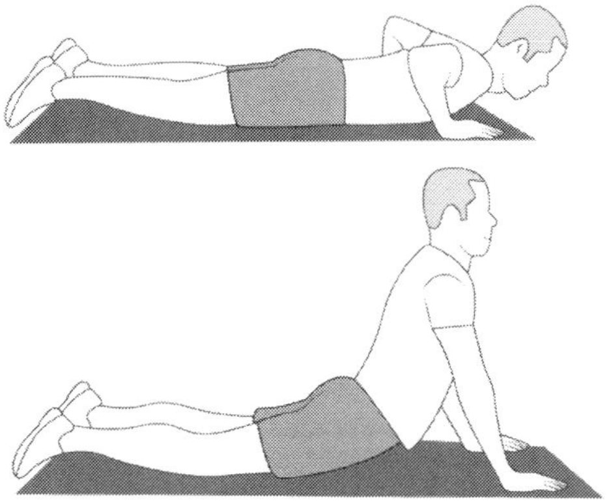

Exercise: Bird Dogs

Body Part: Low Back, Core, Abs, Hamstrings, Glutes

Benefit: Helps with lower back injury recovery, strengthens multiple core muscles

How To: Start on your knees and hands, with hands just under your shoulders and knees, even with your hips. Slowly raise one arm and the opposite leg simultaneously, pointing both forward and backward, respectively. Hold for 2-3 seconds, then slowly return to the original position. Alternate sides and do this 10-12 times.

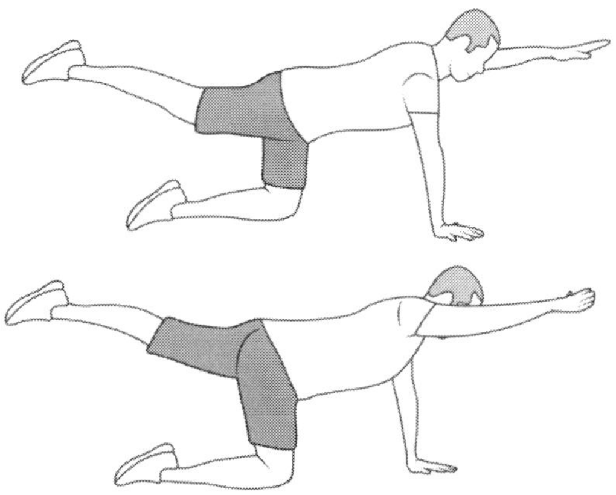

Exercise: Standing Hip Abductions

Body Part: Hips

Benefit: Strengthens hips and helps balance.

How To: Standing straight with your eyes forward, grab the back top of a chair to steady yourself. Place your free hand on your hip and slowly move your outside leg away from your body. Hold your leg out for 1-2 seconds and slowly return to the original position. Do this 8-10 times each leg.

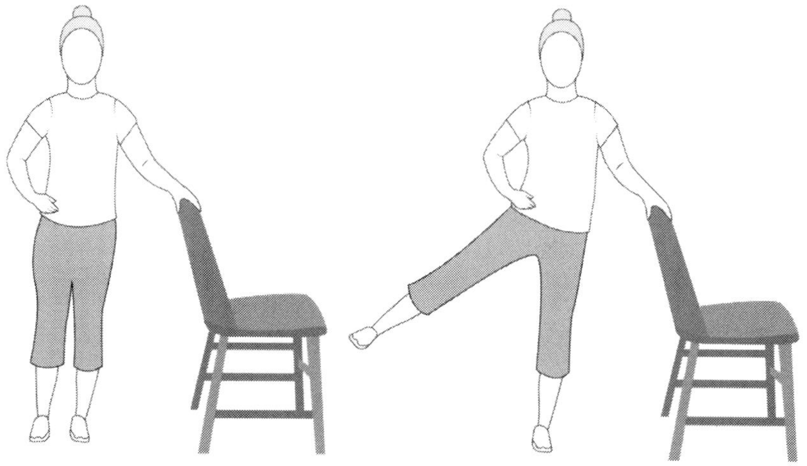

Exercise: Hip Hinges

Body Part: Hips, Abs

Benefit: Strengthens and creates flexibility in hips.

How To: Standing straight with eyes forward and feet hip-width apart, place your hands on your hips. Slowly hinge forward from the hips, keeping your legs and back straight, and bend to about 45-90 degrees. Then, slowly return to the original position. Do this 10-12 times.

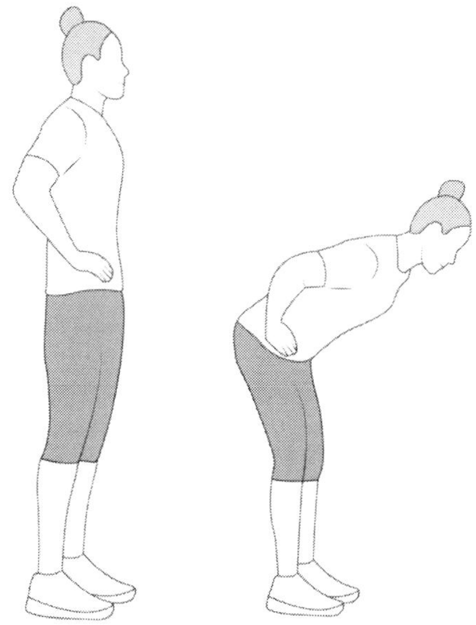

Exercise: Hip Swings

Body Part: Hips, Legs, Abs

Benefit: Strengthens and creates flexibility in hips.

How To: Standing straight with your eyes forward and feet hip-width apart, place your free hand on your hip and the other hand on the top of a chair. Slowly swing one leg forward while keeping the other leg firmly planted on the floor. Slowly return (do not hold) to the original position. Do this 8-10 times each leg.

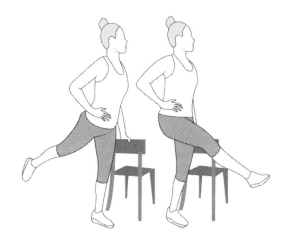

Exercise: Chair Squats

Body Part: Glutes, Legs

Benefit: Strengthens butt and leg muscles, balance

How To: Standing in front of a chair with feet shoulder-width apart, raise your arms out, making them parallel to the floor. Slowly bend your knees and lower your weight into the chair for 1-2 seconds, and then slowly return to the original position. Do this 10-12 times.

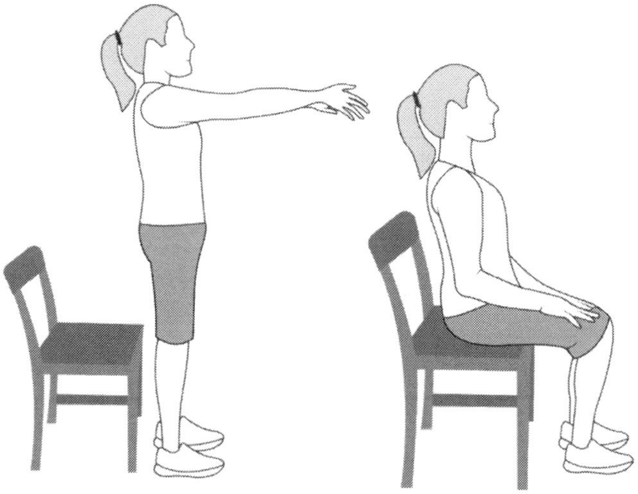

Exercise: Fighter Squats

Body Part: Glutes, Abs, Legs, Back

Benefit: Strengthens multiple muscle groups and provides excellent cardiovascular benefits.

How To: Placing your feet slightly more than shoulder-width apart, squat down until you're almost in a seated position with your butt touching an imaginary chair. Come back up and turn your torso to the right while throwing a left-hand punch. Come back down to the squat position and then do the same thing to the opposite side. Do this 15-20 times.

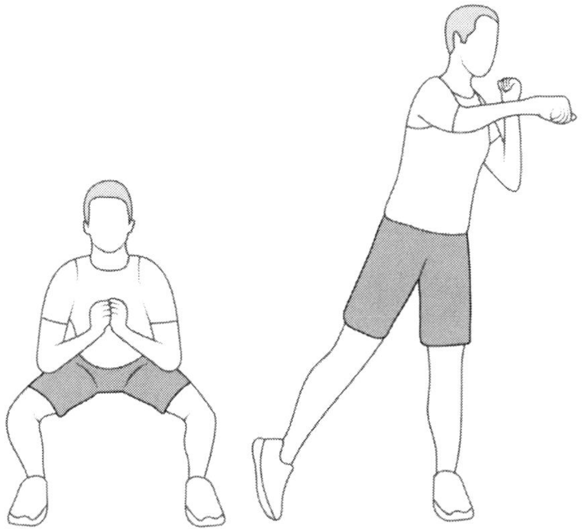

Exercise: Leg Extensions

Body Part: Legs (Hamstrings, Quadriceps), Knees

Benefit: Strengthens and stretches leg muscles

How To: Sitting up straight and back into a chair, plant your feet on the floor shoulder-width apart. Slowly raise one leg until it's parallel to the floor. Then flex your toes back for 1-2 seconds. Slowly come back down and repeat the motion with the other foot. Do this 10-12 times per leg.

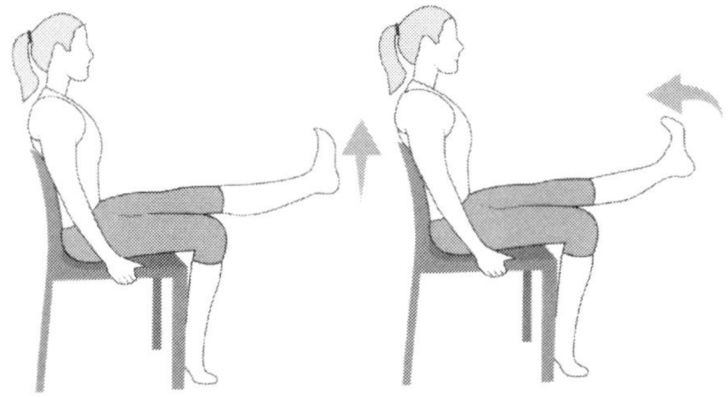

Exercise: Seated Knee Raises

Body Part: Legs (Quadriceps), Hips

Benefit: Strengthens quads, flexibility in the hips

How To: Sitting straight on a chair, with eyes forward and feet less than hip-length apart, slowly raise one knee as high as you can. Slowly come back down and make the same motion with your opposite leg. Continue this 15-20 times.

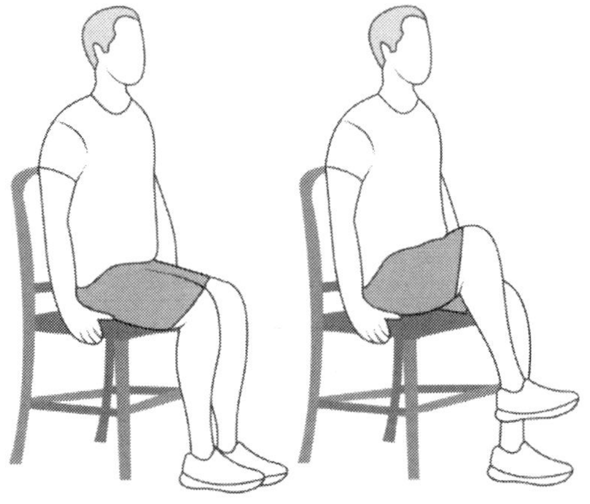

Exercise: Mini Lunges

Body Part: Legs, Hips, Low Back, Knees, Glutes

Benefit: Strengthens the lower body, helps with balance

How To: Standing straight up with eyes forward and feet shoulder-width apart, stand on the outside back of a chair. Using your left hand, grab the top of the chair for stability. Slowly lunge forward with your right leg, bending your knee to no more than 45 degrees. Slowly return to the original position. Do this 10 times per leg.

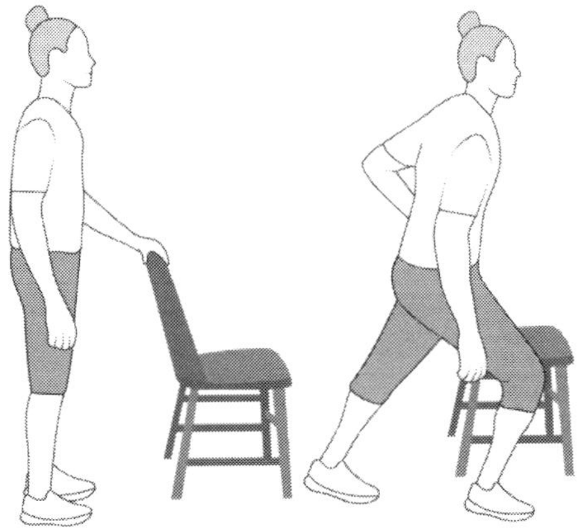

Exercise: Step Ups

Body Part: Legs (Quads), Glutes, Knees

Benefit: Strengthens legs, helps with balance

How To: Standing near the stairs, place your inside hand on a railing or wall for balance. With one leg, slowly step up to the first stair and bring your other leg up to the step, ensuring both feet are securely on the step. Slowly bring the second (trail) leg back down to the floor and then the first leg. Make sure both feet are secure before another rep. Do this 10-15 times, and then change your lead leg.

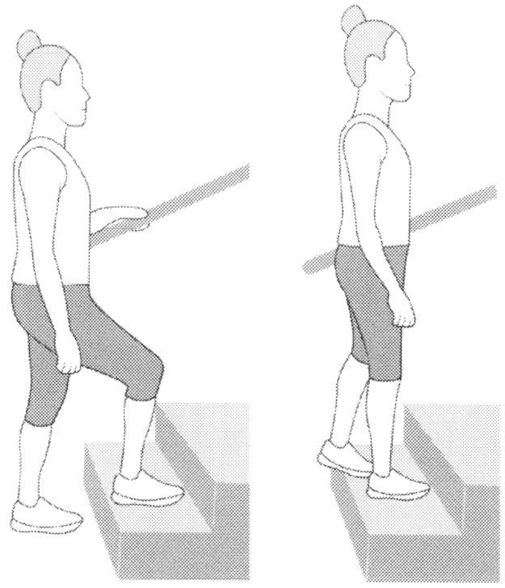

Exercise: Side Lunges

Body Part: Legs (Quads, Hamstrings), Hips

Benefit: Strengthens legs, helps with balance

How To: Standing straight with feet slightly less than shoulder-width apart, place your hands up to your chest (for balance). With eyes forward, slowly pick one leg up slightly off the floor and "lunge" this lead leg to the side. Bending at the knee, keep most of your weight on the bent knee side while keeping the other leg straight and secure. Slowly return to the starting position and repeat with the other leg. Do this 10 times per leg.

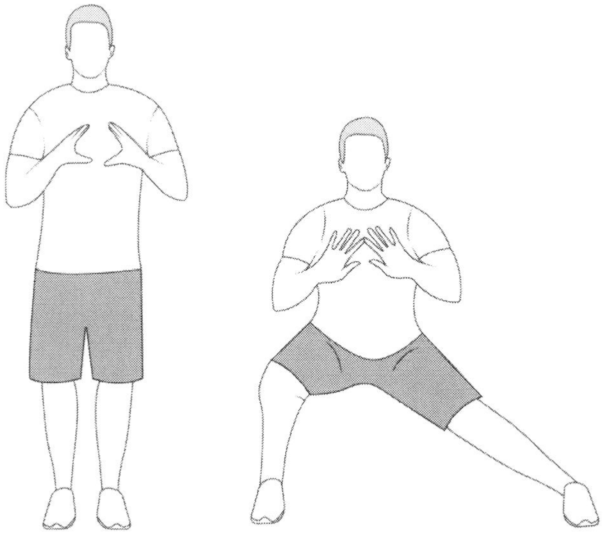

Exercise: Standing Hamstring Curls

Body Part: Hamstrings, Hips

Benefit: Strengthens legs, helps hip flexibility

How To: Standing straight up with feet hip-width apart and eyes forward, hold the back of a chair with both hands for balance. Slowly bend one leg until it's parallel to the floor. Hold for 1-2 seconds, then slowly return your leg to the original position. Do this 10-12 times per leg.

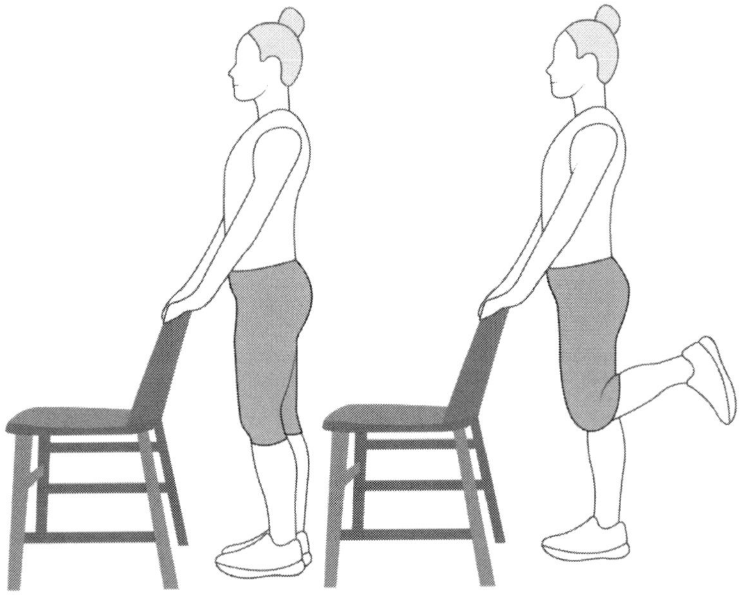

Exercise: Hamstring "Mule" Kickbacks

Body Part: Hamstrings, Hips, Glutes

Benefit: Strengthens legs and glutes, helps hip flexibility

How To: Standing straight up with feet hip-width apart and eyes forward, hold the back of a chair with both hands for balance. Lift one of your feet off the ground and kick it back while engaging your core and glutes. Be sure your motion remains smooth and not jerky. Return your foot to the original position. Do this 10 times with each leg.

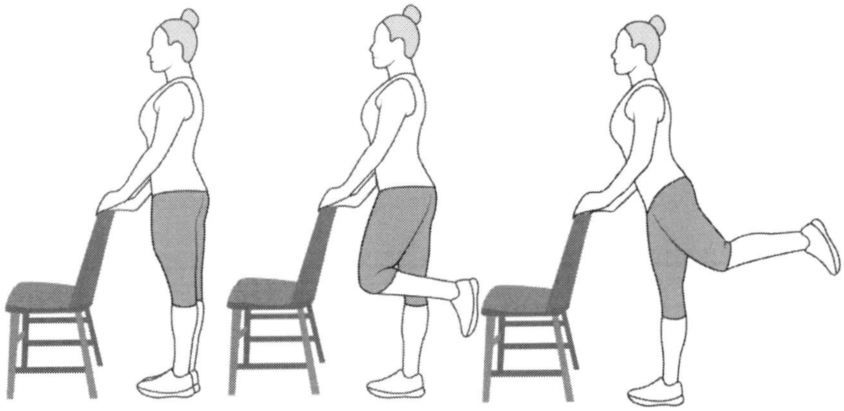

Exercise: Chair Calf Raises

Body Part: Legs (Calves), Glutes, Ankles

Benefit: Isolates and strengthens calves, helps with balance

How To: Standing straight up with feet hip-width apart and eyes forward, hold the back of a chair (or on a wall) with both hands for balance. Slowly raise up on both feet's toes until you can't go any higher. Hold for 1-2 seconds and slowly return to the original position. Do this 10-12 times.

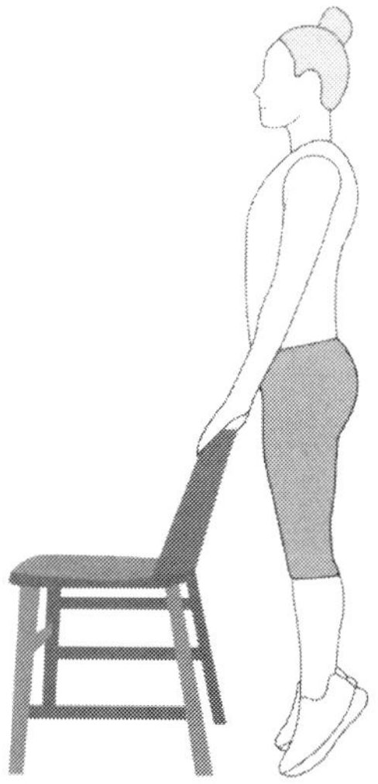

Exercise: Weighted Calf Raises

Body Part: Legs (Calves), Glutes, Ankles

Benefit: Isolates and strengthens calves, helps with balance

How To: Taking light dumbbells in both hands, stand straight with feet hip-width apart and eyes forward. Slowly raise up on both feet's toes until you can't go any higher. Hold for 1-2 seconds and slowly return to the original position. Do this 10-12 times. Use this exercise as a "graduation" from Chair Calf Raises.

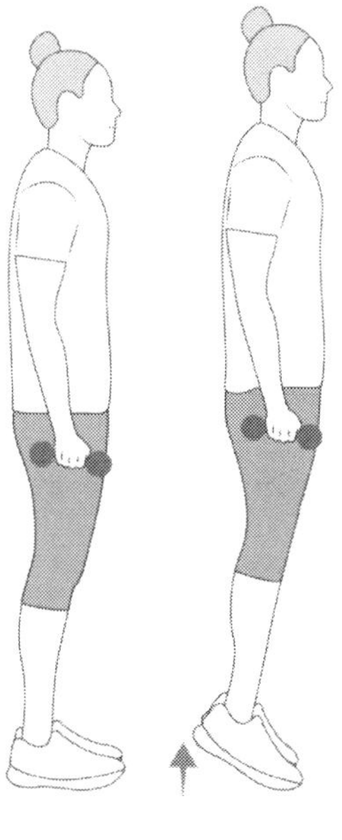

Full Body Strength Exercises

Exercise: Mountain Climbers

Body Part: Shoulders, Abs, Legs (Quads), Hips, Glutes

Benefit: Works multiple muscles, helps balance and coordination, and improves cardiovascular health.

How To: Standing with your feet shoulder-width apart, reach up with one arm (as if climbing), and simultaneously bring up the opposite knee/leg to about 45 degrees. Return to the original position and promptly perform the same motion with the other arm and leg. Be sure your movements are smooth and not jerky. Do this 12-15 times.

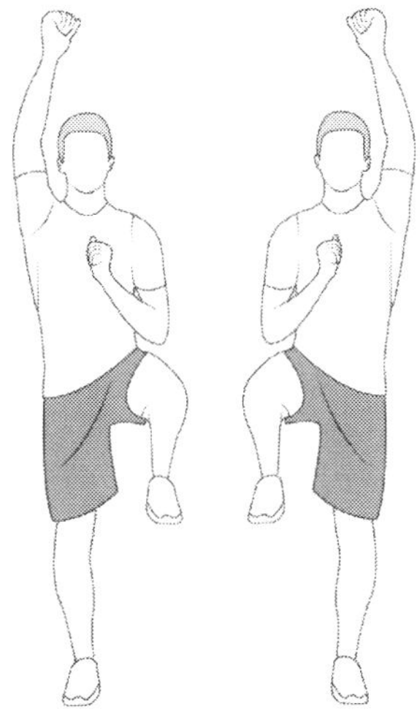

Exercise: Lunging Bicep Curl

Body Part: Biceps, Legs (Quads, Hamstrings), Glutes

Benefit: Works multiple muscles, helps balance.

How To: Take light dumbbells in both hands, stand straight with your legs together and your eyes forward. Simultaneously and slowly lunge one leg forward while bringing up both hands and weights in a curl motion towards your chest. Then, slowly return both your arms and first leg to the original position. Do this 10-12 times.

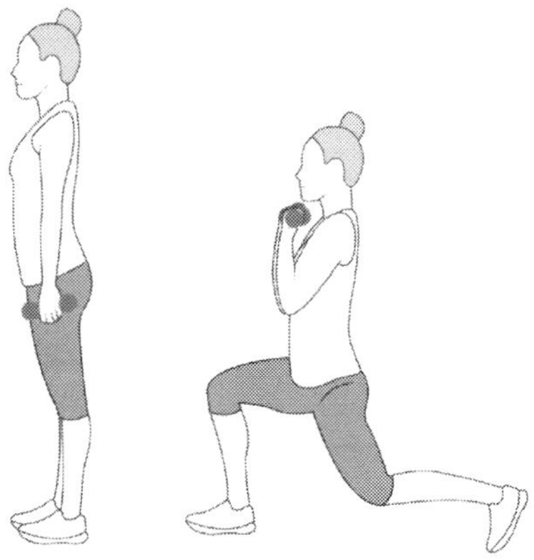

Exercise: Single Leg Forward Reach

Body Part: Shoulders, Core, Glutes, Hips

Benefit: Works multiple muscles, helps balance and coordination

How To: Standing straight with your feet hip-width apart, slowly bend one knee and bring your leg backward. Simultaneously raise both hands outward as you bend forward, keeping your weight on one leg. Slowly return to the original position and alternate legs. Do this 10 times. NOTE: Please have a chair handy for this one for additional balance if needed.

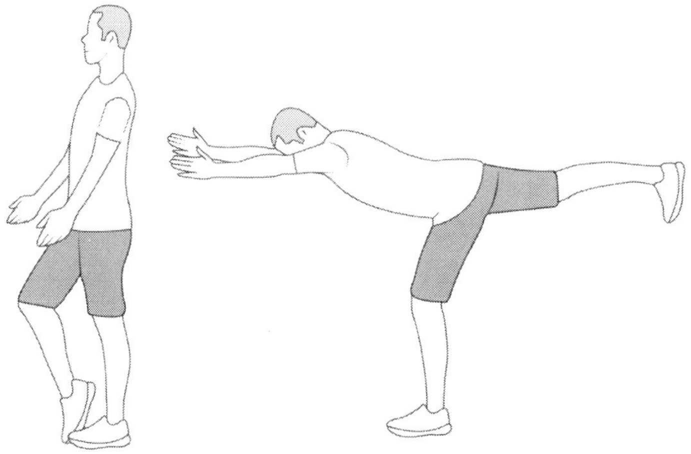

Exercise: Squatting Reaches

Body Part: Legs (Quads, Hamstrings), Glutes, Shoulders

Benefit: Works multiple muscles, helps balance and coordination

How To: Standing straight with your feet shoulder-width apart and eyes forward, slowly lowering your butt to a 45-degree angle while raising your arms above your head. Hold the squat for 1-2 seconds, then slowly return to the original position. Do this 10-12 times.

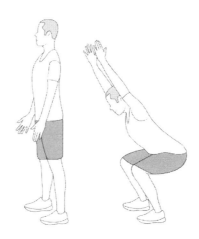

Stretching & Warm-up Exercises

Because stretching is more about warming up your muscles than strengthening them, stretching is a great time to focus on breathing, relaxing, and preparing your mind for your exercises. Stretching can be a very meditative activity. In fact, the stretching and warming-up portions of your workout can even be used as a workout itself. You won't be as many calories, but it will get you moving, which is half the battle.

Just like with the strength exercises, you can do many of these stretches, standing up or seated.

Exercise: Rolling Neck

Body Part: Neck

Benefit: Stretches neck muscles

How To: Standing straight up with shoulders square and arms at your side, slowly bring your head forward and slowly roll it to the left (or right) until you've made one full rotation. Keep slowly rolling and continue this motion to the chosen side for 10 repetitions. Then, slowly come to a stop and reverse direction for another 10 reps.

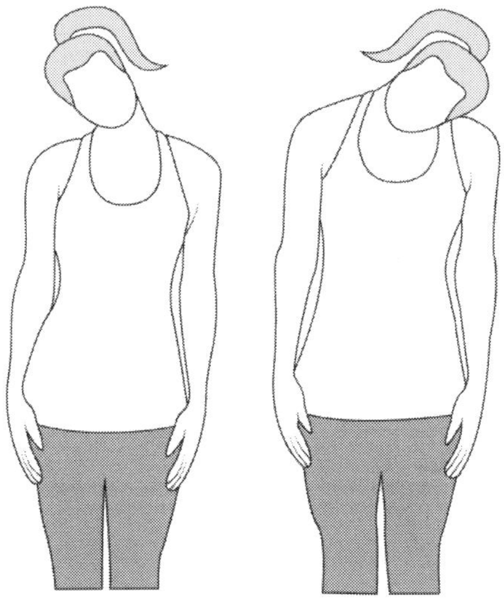

Exercise: The Ostrich Neck

Body Part: Neck

Benefit: Stretches neck muscles

How To: Standing straight with shoulders square, eyes forward, and arms at your side, slowly glide your head back, so your chin feels tucked for 1-2 seconds. Slowly move your head forward and away from your shoulders. Return to the original position and do this 10-12 times.

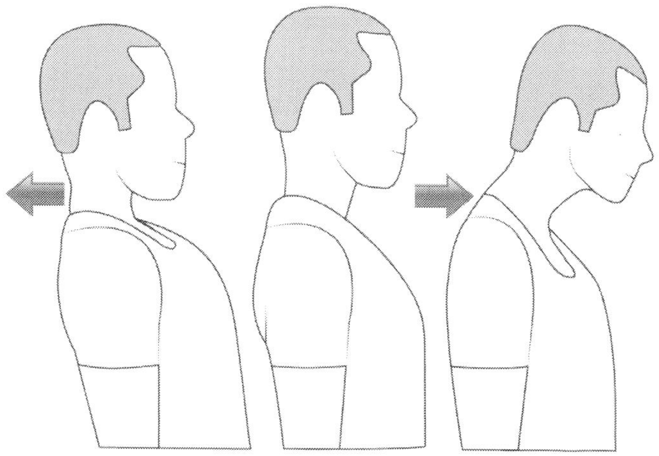

Exercise: Neck Extensions

Body Part: Neck

Benefit: Stretches neck muscles

How To: Standing straight with shoulders square and arms at your side, slowly bring your head back until your chin points up. Hold this for 5 seconds and slowly bring your head forward, tucking your chin to your chest for 5 seconds. Repeat this 10-12 times.

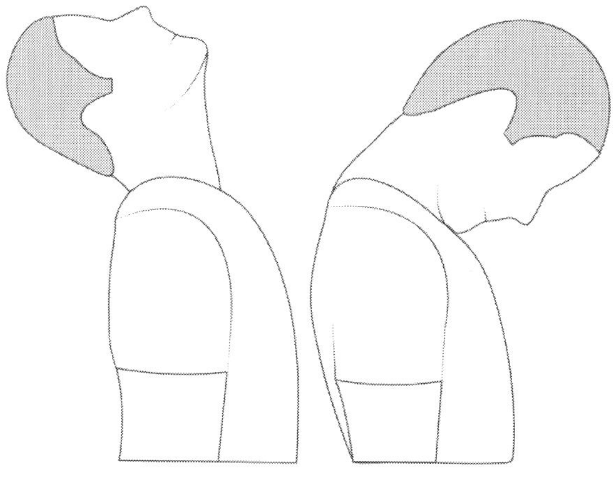

Exercise: Relaxed Arm Shakeouts

Body Part: Arms, Wrists, Hands

Benefit: Loosens arms and wrists and eliminates tension

How To: Standing (or sitting) straight with shoulders relaxed and arms at your side, begin loosely shaking your hands and arms. Open and close your hands to loosen up your fingers while shaking. Do this for about 10-15 seconds.

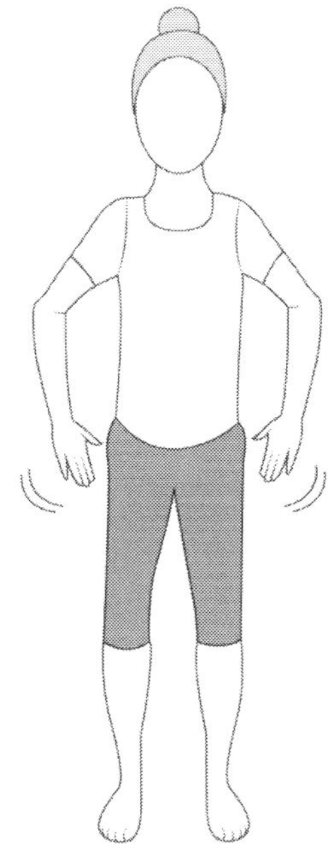

Exercise: Wrist Stretches

Body Part: Wrist, Forearm

Benefit: Stretches wrists and forearms and helps with carpal tunnel issues.

How To: Standing straight with your shoulders square, extend both arms in front of you and take one hand into the other, fingers pointed down, palm facing you. Slowly pull back on the one hand for 5 seconds. Now turn that same hand so the palm is facing away from you. Fingers remain down. Pull your fingers back for 5 seconds. Do this with both wrists.

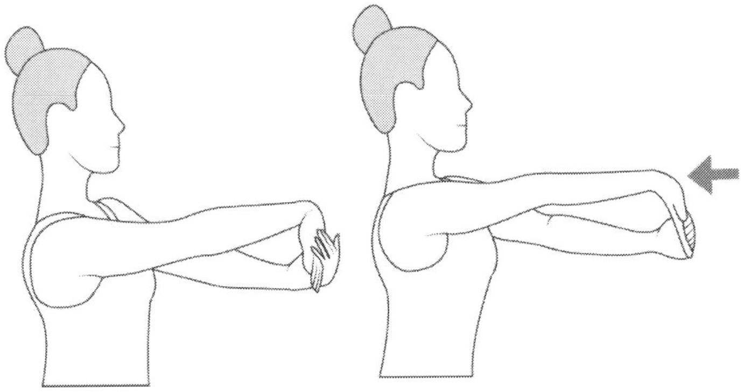

Exercise: Bicep Stretches

Body Part: Bicep, Shoulders

Benefit: Stretches arms (biceps),

How To: Sitting on the floor with knees bent, slowly lean back and place your hands flat behind you. Very slowly, scoot your butt forward until you feel a slight stretch in your arms. Breath in/out deeply and hold for about 10 seconds, then return to the original position. Do this 5-7 times.

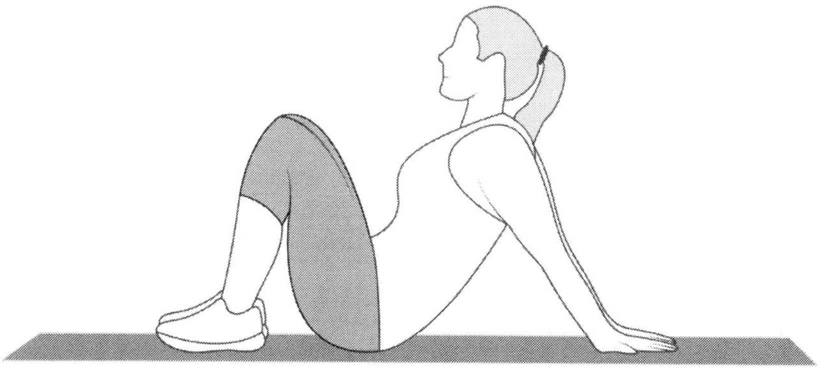

Exercise: Overhead Tricep Stretches

Body Part: Tricep, Shoulders, Upper Back

Benefit: Stretches and relaxes arms, shoulders, and back

How To: Standing straight with eyes forward, place one arm behind your head and take hold of your elbow with the other hand. Slowly pull your elbow back until you feel mild tension in your arm and shoulder. Do this 5-10 seconds and 5-7 times per arm.

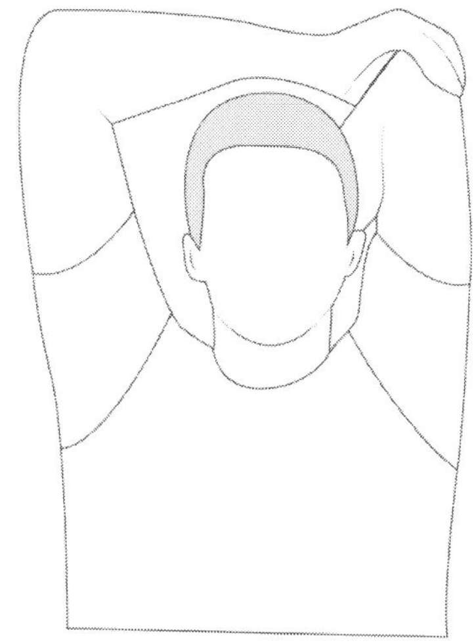

Exercise: Prayer Stretches

Body Part: Arms, Shoulders, Elbows, Wrists

Benefit: Stretches and relaxes muscles and joints

How To: Sitting straight with shoulder square and eyes forward, bring your hands together in a prayer-like position. Push your palms together slightly until you feel mild tension in your arms. Then, slowly bring your hands up, even to your face. Hold for 5 seconds and return to the original position. Do this 8-10 times.

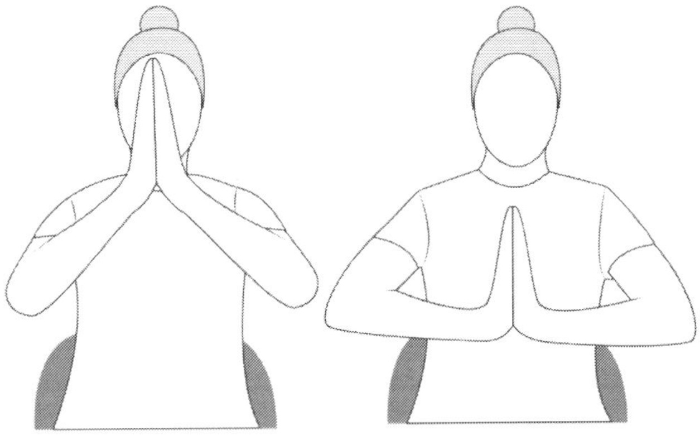

Exercise: Chest and Arm Stretches

Body Part: Chest, Biceps, Shoulders

Benefit: Stretches multiple upper body muscles

How To: Standing parallel to the side of a wall, with feet together, shoulders square, and eyes forward, bring your arm back behind you against the wall. Slowly turn your body slightly away from the wall while keeping your palm flat. Once you feel mild tension, hold that for 5 seconds and return to the original position. Do this 5 times and switch arms.

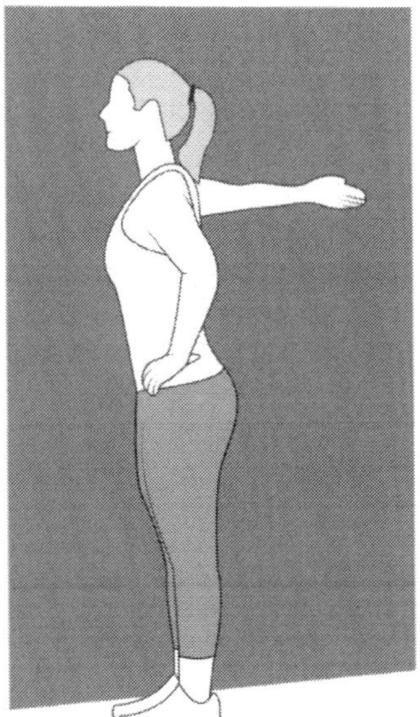

Exercise: Reaching for the Sky

Body Part: Shoulders, Upper Back

Benefit: Stretches shoulders and back, helps core breathing

How To: Sitting straight with feet flat and eyes forward, take your hands and join them together by interlocking your fingers. Slowly bring your hands up and turn your palms toward the ceiling. Hold for 5-10 seconds and slowly return to the original position. Do this 5 times.

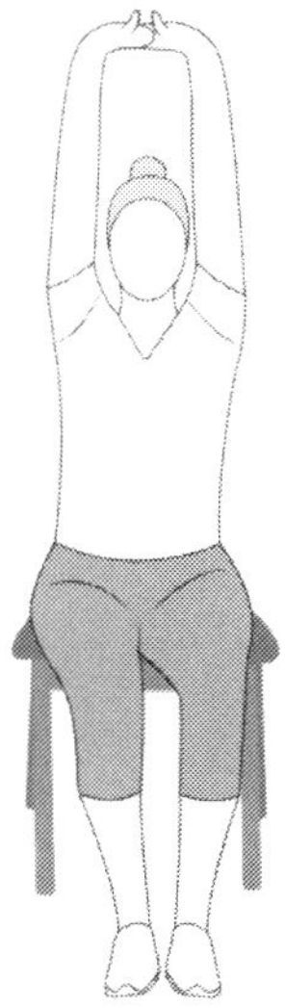

Exercise: One Arm Hugs

Body Part: Shoulders, Upper Back, Chest

Benefit: Stretches multiple upper body muscles at once.

How To: Sitting on the floor with your legs crossed, shoulders square, and eyes forward, bring one arm across your chest above your shoulder. With your other arm, gently pull your upper arm back (above the elbow) until you feel mild tension in your upper arm. Hold this for 10 seconds, then change arms. Do this 5 times per arm. Note: this is an exercise you can also do while standing.

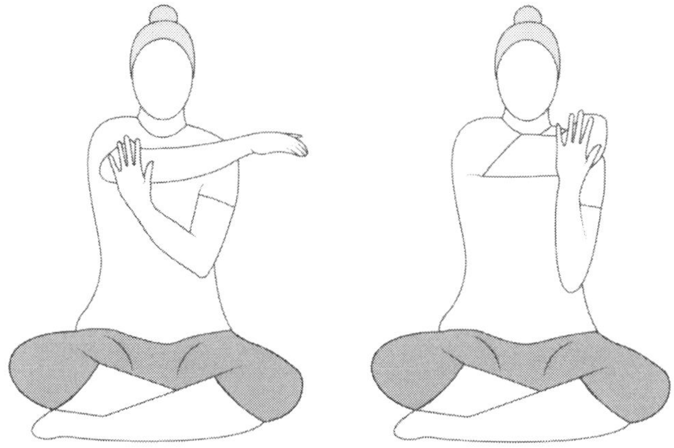

Exercise: Shoulder Pulls

Body Part: Shoulders, Upper Back

Benefit: Stretches and reduces tension in shoulders and back

How To: Standing straight with shoulders square, feet together, and eyes forward, slowly inhale deeply and bring your shoulders backward while slowly pushing out your chest. Hold this for 3-5 seconds. Exhale and return to the original position. Do this 10 times.

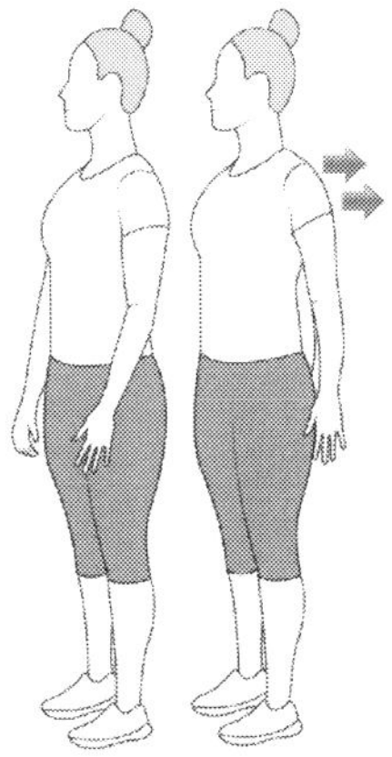

Exercise: Marching in Place

Body Part: Legs, Arms

Benefit: Good warm-up for strength exercises, helps balance

How To: Standing straight with shoulders square, feet together, and eyes forward, slowly begin marching. Exaggerate your arms and legs, so your hands come as high as your face and knees to 45 degrees. Pick up the tempo slightly as your march, but stay balanced. Focus on good breathing and marching mechanics. Do this for 30 seconds.

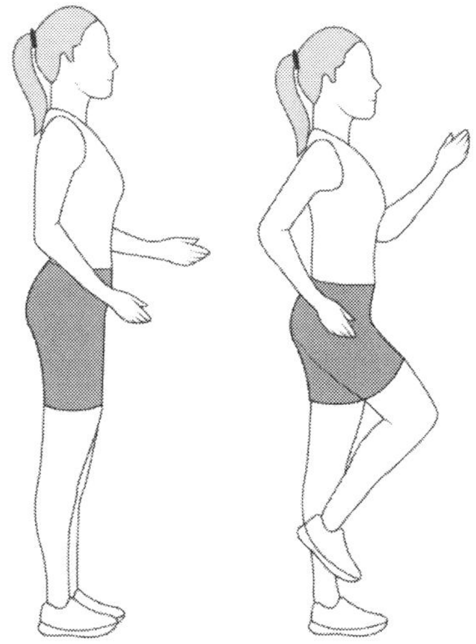

Exercise: The Sideways Shuffle

Body Part: Legs

Benefit: Good warm-up for strength exercises, helps balance

How To: Standing straight with feet slightly greater than shoulder-width apart, knees bent slightly and eyes forward, slowly shuffle to one side. To "shuffle," bring one foot next to the other, never crossing your feet. If you have enough space, do this 3-5 times to the right and 3-5 times to the left. Keep going back and forth for 30 seconds.

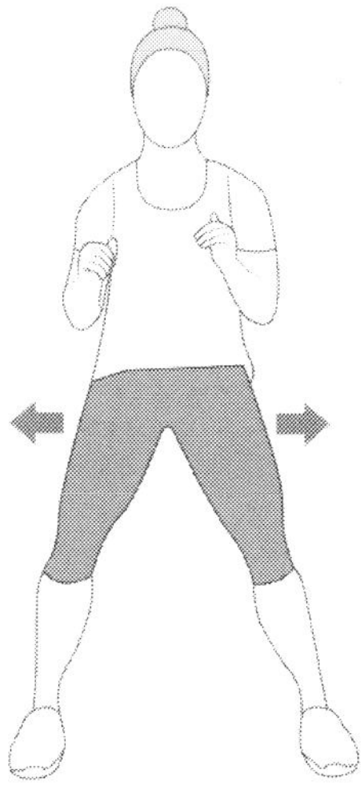

Exercise: Smooth Twists

Body Part: Core, Upper Body, Hips, Spine

Benefit: Relaxes torso and spine stability

How To: Standing straight with shoulders square, feet hip-width apart, and eyes forward, place hands on your hips. Slowly and smoothly rotate your torso and head to the right while keeping your feet firmly planted. Stop when you feel a slight tension and return to the original position. Then rotate to the left in the same fashion. Be very careful not to over-twist. Do this for about 30 seconds.

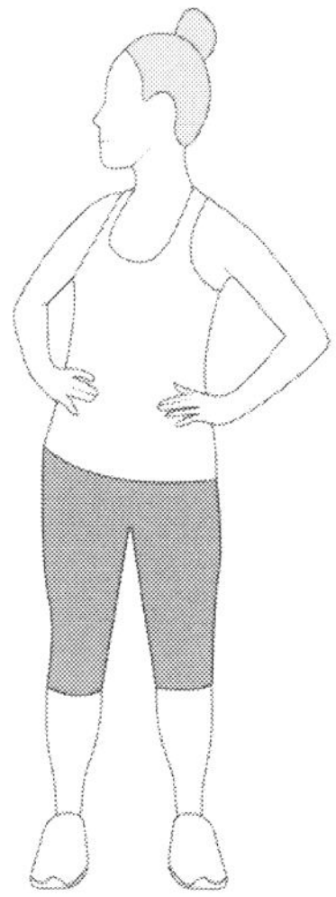

Exercise: Overhead Side Stretches

Body Part: Hips, Shoulders, Back

Benefit: Stretches shoulders and core, helps balance

How To: Standing straight with feet slightly greater than shoulder-width apart and eyes forward, reach up to the ceiling with both arms. Place your palms together and slowly lean to the side, keeping your feet stationary. When you reach about 25 degrees, slowly come back up and repeat to the opposite side. Do this 5-10 times per side.

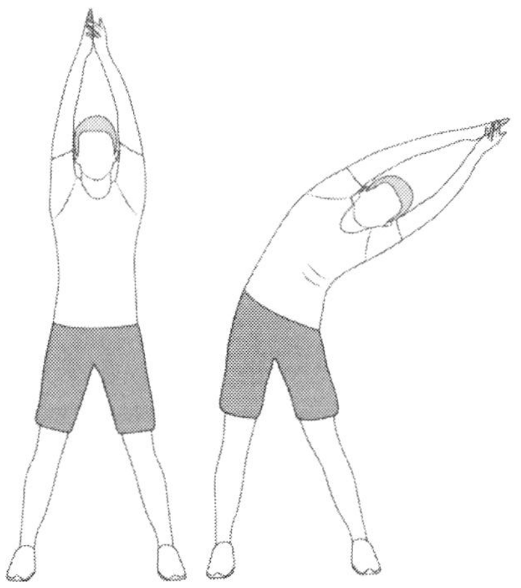

Exercise: Hip Circles

Body Part: Hips, Spine

Benefit: Stretches hips, helps with balance and spine

How To: Standing straight with feet shoulder-width apart and eyes forward, place your hands on your hips. Slowly and gently start to rotate your hips around in a circle. Do this 5 times to one side, then gradually stop and reverse directions for 5 times.

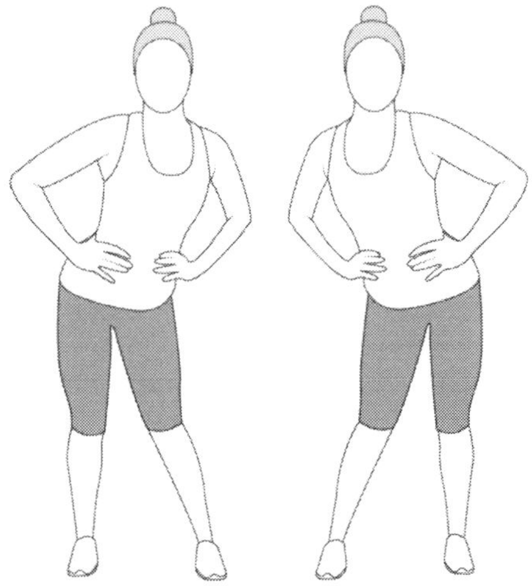

Exercise: Child's Pose

Body Part: Shoulders, Back, Legs

Benefit: Helps stretch and relax multiple muscles

How To: Starting with both knees on the floor and sitting back on your hunches, slowly bring your face towards the floor and lean forward, bringing your hands up above your head. Place your hands on the floor and extend them away slowly from your body. When you feel a mild stretch in your shoulders, hold for 5 seconds, then release the stretch. Do this 8-10 times.

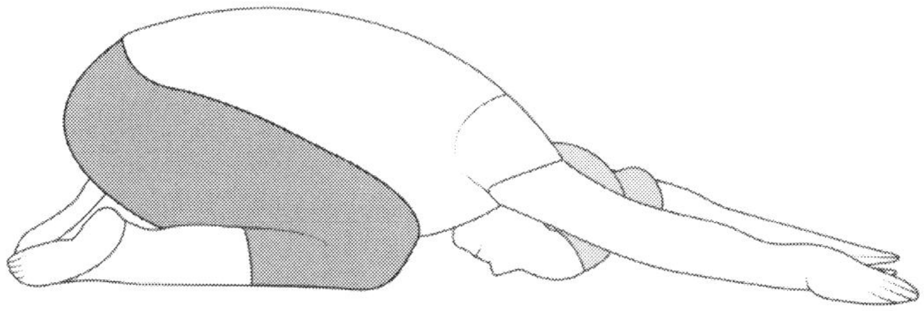

Exercise: Cat-Cows

Body Part: Back, Neck, Core

Benefit: Stretches neck, core, and spine and helps breathing

How To: Starting with both knees and hands on the floor, place your knees hip-width apart and your hands shoulder-width apart. Slowly arch your back into a scared cat-like position while relaxing your neck downward. Hold for 3-5 seconds and slowly return to the cow-like position bringing your head back up with eyes forward. Do this 5-7 times slowly.

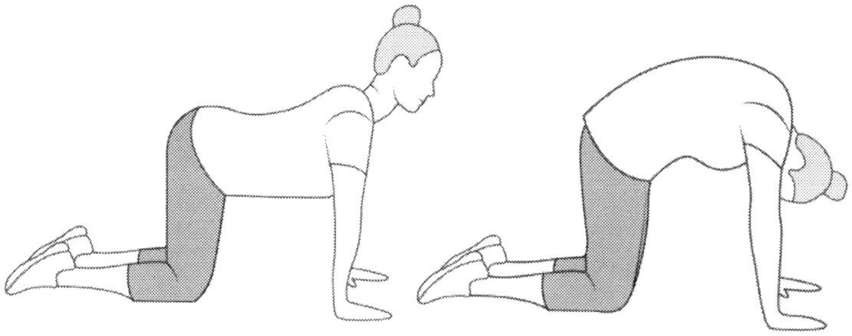

Exercise: Single Knee to Chest Stretches

Body Part: Lower Back, Glutes

Benefit: Stretches lower back and glutes

How To: Lying with your head, back, and legs flat on the floor, slowly bring up one leg and grab it with both hands behind your knee. Slowly pull your leg towards your chest until you feel a mild stretch. Hold this for 5 seconds and loosen the stretch. Do this 5 times each leg.

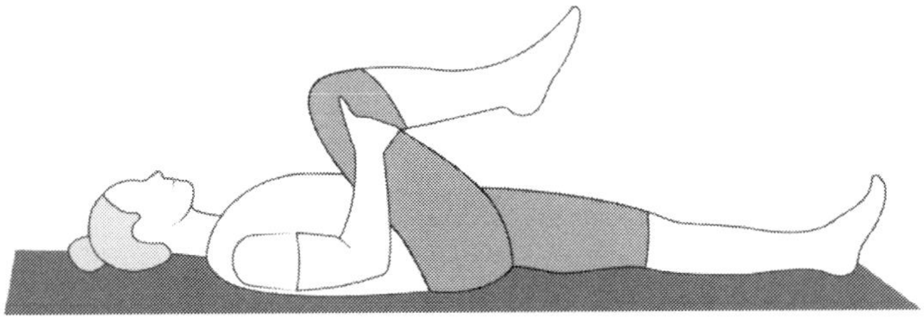

Exercise: Knees to Chest Stretches

Body Part: Lower Back, Glutes

Benefit: Stretches lower back and glutes

How To: This is similar to the single knee to chest stretch but with both knees. Lying with your head, back and legs flat on the floor, slowly bring up both legs and grasp with both hands above your knee. Slowly pull your legs towards your chest until you feel a mild stretch. Hold this for 5 seconds and loosen the stretch. Do this 10 times.

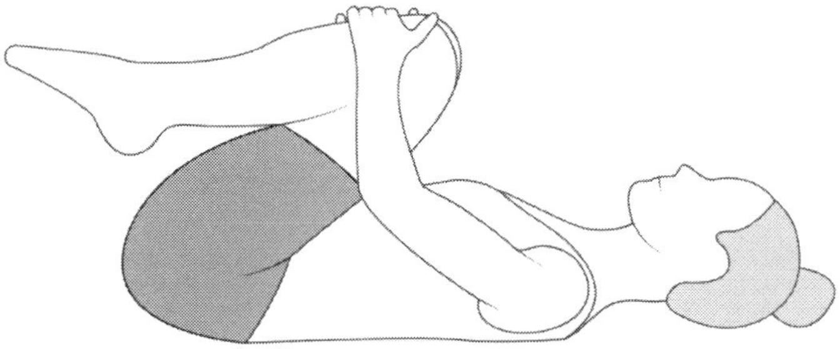

Exercise: Standing Quad Stretches

Body Part: Legs (Quadriceps)

Benefit: Stretches quadriceps muscles

How To: Standing behind a chair, with feet hip-width apart, use one hand to balance on the back of the chair. Then, slowly bring the opposite leg backward and up and grab the top of your foot, pulling it into your glutes until you feel a mild stretch. Hold this position for 5-10 seconds and do this 5 times per leg.

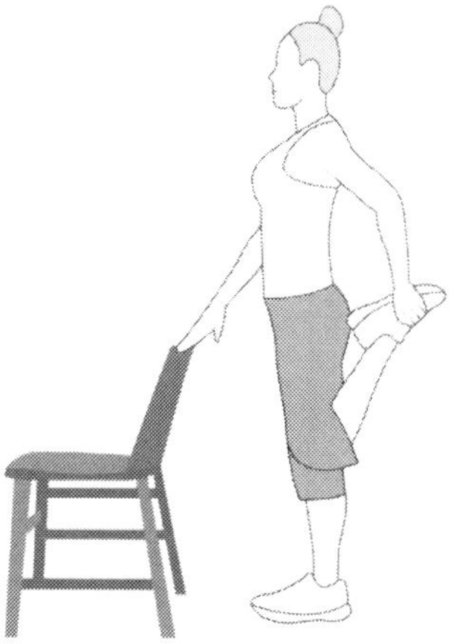

Exercise: Seated Hamstring Stretches

Body Part: Legs (Hamstrings)

Benefit: Stretches hamstring muscles

How To: Sitting on a chair towards the mid/front, place one leg straight out and the other bent at 45 degrees. Locking your straight leg, with your hands resting on your bent leg, slowly move forward until you feel a mild stretch. Keep your back straight. Hold this for 5-10 seconds and switch legs. Do this 5 times per leg.

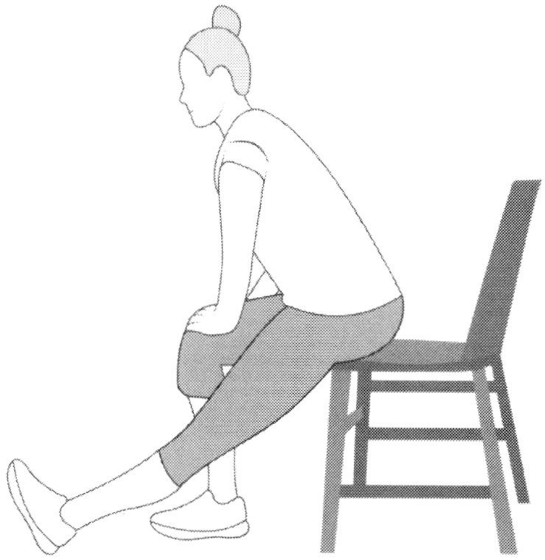

Exercise: Calf Wall Stretches

Body Part: Legs (Calves), Glutes

Benefit: Stretches calf muscles and glutes

How To: Place your hands flat on a wall and extend one leg behind you until it's completely straight with the heal up and toes down. Slowly bring your heel down to the floor to feel your calf stretch. Hold the stretch for about 5-10 seconds, then slowly raise your heel back up to remove the tension. Do this 5 times per leg.

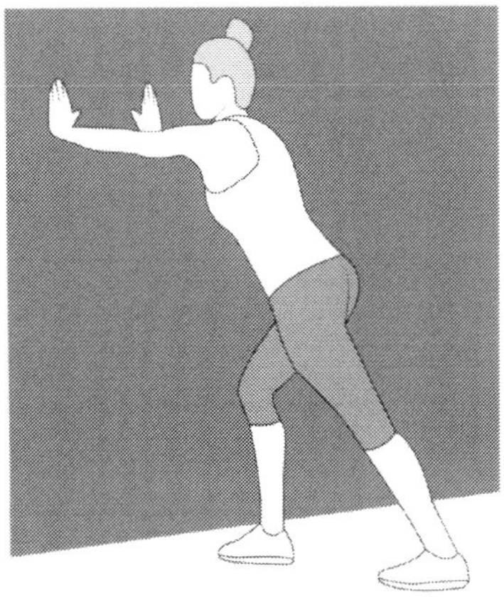

Exercise: Seated Glute Stretches (Mom's Favorite)

Body Part: Glutes, Hips

Benefit: Stretches glutes and helps hip flexibility

How To: Sitting upright on a chair, place both feet flat on the floor and then cross one leg over the opposite knee. Grasp your knee with both hands and slowly pull it forward towards your shoulder while leaning slightly forward towards your knee for 5-10 seconds. Do this 5 times per leg.

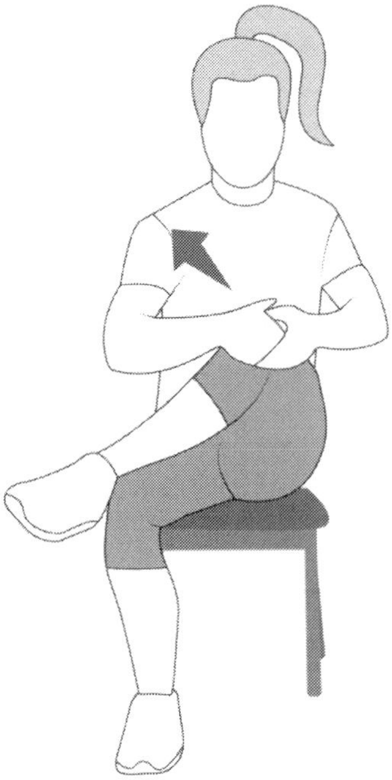

Exercise: Knee Circles

Body Part: Knees

Benefit: Flexibility in knees, helps with balance

How To: Standing with your feet and knees together and hands on your knees, slowly and gently rotate your knees together simultaneously in a circle. Be sure to keep from slouching your back. Do this 5-10 times in one direction, then reverse directions.

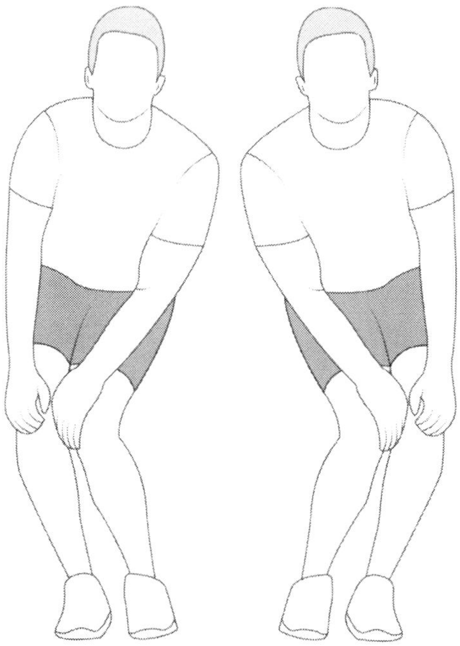

Exercise: Butterflies

Body Part: Hips, Hamstring, Groin

Benefit: Flexibility in hips helps with posture

How To: Sitting with the bottoms of your feet together, hold your ankles and relax your shoulders. Slowly arch your back while pushing your chest slightly forward while also leaning forward. Feel the stretch in your inside legs for 5-10 seconds. Then, slowly release the stretch and repeat this motion 10 times.

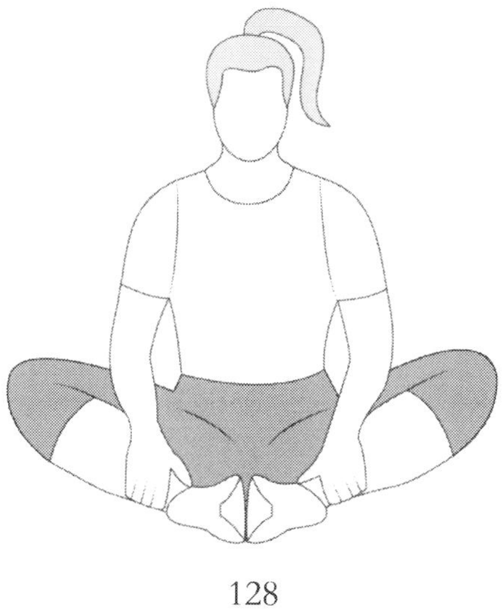

Exercise: Ankle Pumps

Body Part: Ankles

Benefit: Stretches ankles, and calves, helps balance

How To: Sitting on the floor with a foam roller or rolled-up towel, extend one leg on top of the roller and bend the other to about 45 degrees. Keeping your bent leg's foot planted, start pointing your toe outwards for 1-2 seconds and then back towards you for 1-2 seconds. Do this 10-12 times per ankle.

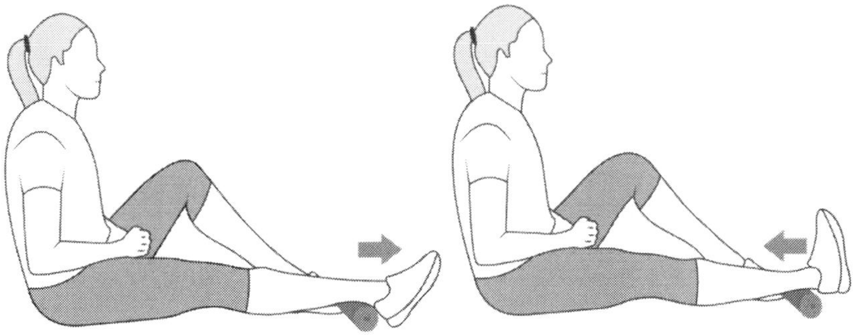

Exercise: Ankle Circles

Body Part: Ankles

Benefit: Flexibility in ankles, helps with balance

How To: Sitting back in a chair, with your hands on the sides, cross one leg over the opposite leg over the knee. Slowly rotate your ankle in a large circle for 5-10 repetitions. Reverse direction for 5-10 more circles. Alternate legs and do the same number of rotations each way.

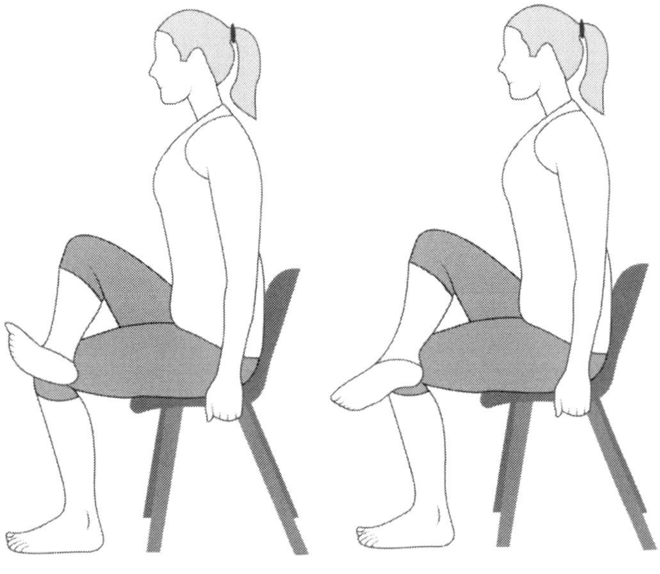

Chapter 9
Give Me Strength Workouts

"Sweat is just fat crying."

- Anonymous

This chapter contains eleven different and highly effective workout routines. Each one has a purpose. You can use them as a stand-alone workout or replace any exercise with any on the list in Chapter 8 (per category) based on your comfort level and pain tolerance for that exercise.

The beauty of the routines in this book is that they're fully customizable. Essentially, there are a limitless number of workouts available. So if you see an exercise you'd like to remove and replace, you have that flexibility. Remember that the comprehensive list of exercises in Chapter 8 is like an ala carte menu to pick and choose the exercises that work for you.

THE WORKOUTS

Here is the list of the 11 workouts:

- Foundations (Beginner) - Full Body Workout
- Next Steps (Intermediate) - Full Body Workout
- Tip-Top 10 (Advanced) - Full Body Workout
- Balance 5 - Core Workout
- Balance 7 - Core Workout
- Quickie Cardio - Mini Full Body Workout
- Pain Relief Workouts:
- Neck/Back/Shoulders
- Sciatica/Back

- Knees/Hips/Ankles
- Wrist, Elbows
- Give Me Strength Special - Full Body Workout

Note: For a detailed "how to" of each exercise, please refer to Chapter 8.

We've already discussed this extensively in previous chapters, but I cannot stress it enough. Please remember that good posture (form) and breathing are essential when exercising. These things are much more important than the amount of weight you lift and the number of repetitions you can do. Be conscious of it as you near the end of your workouts, as that is when bad form starts to creep in when you're tired.Another essential tip going into the actual workouts is to stay hydrated. We also covered this in earlier chapters, but it's another critical part of maximizing your ability to sustain through the entire workout. So keep a water bottle close by and take some swigs if you ever feel thirsty.

Stretching and Warm-Ups - The Start of Each Workout

Stretching and warming up are an integral part of your pre-workout routines. The following is a simple warm-up and stretching guide or template. This routine should elevate your heart rate slightly and prepare your muscles and joints as you move into the workouts.

As a template, you can substitute other stretches from chapter 8 if different stretches feel better to you. The idea here is to get your whole body prepped, your heart rate up, and blood flowing faster than your resting levels.

You can also substitute other mild cardio exercises that help accomplish this. Even simple chores around the house will work (my mom would say). And remember, "any movement is exercise." Just be mindful that we don't want to be too tired at this stage. We want to start getting our minds and bodies ready for the next step…the workout.

Stretching and Warm-up: 5-10 mins

1. Marching in Place (1 min)

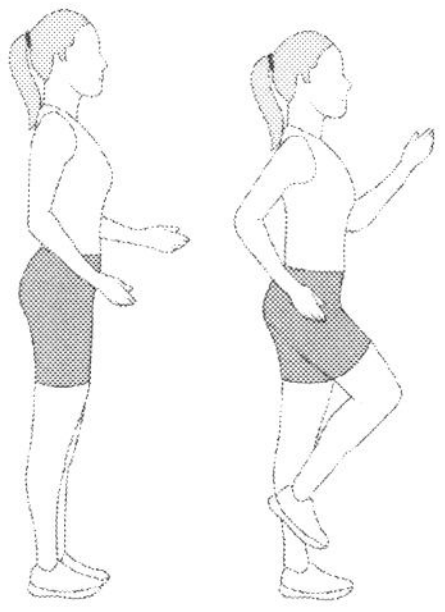

2. Rolling Neck (15-30 secs)

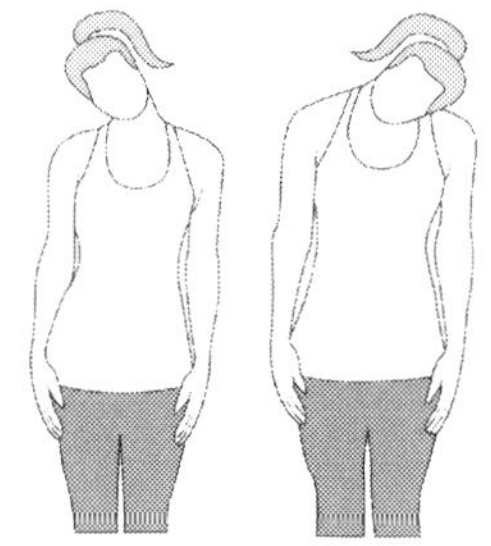

3. Arm Swings (15-30 secs)

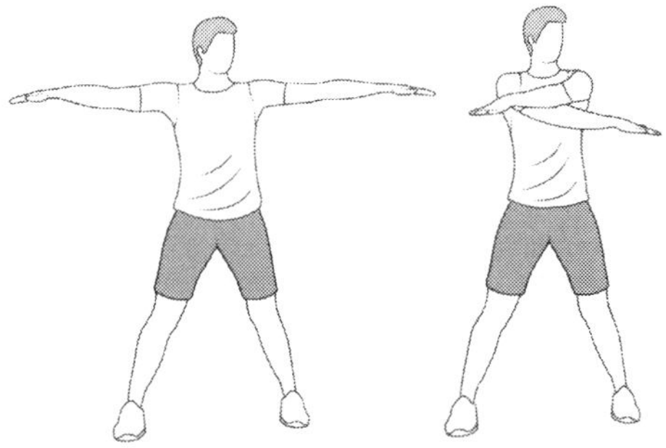

4. Sideways Shuffle (1 min)

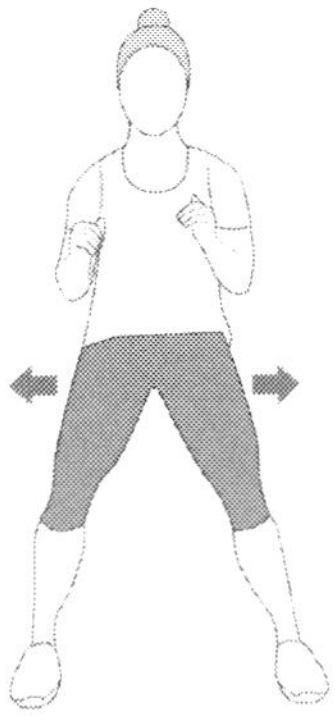

5. Relaxed Arm Shakeouts (15-30 secs)

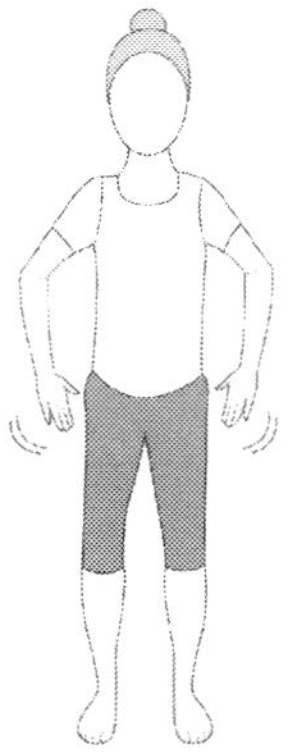

6. Smooth Twists (15-30 secs)

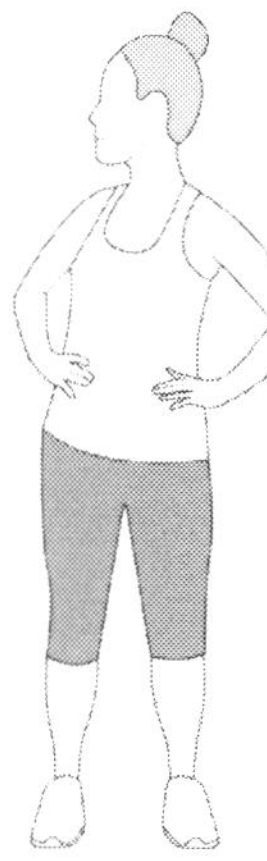

7. Marching in Place (1 min)

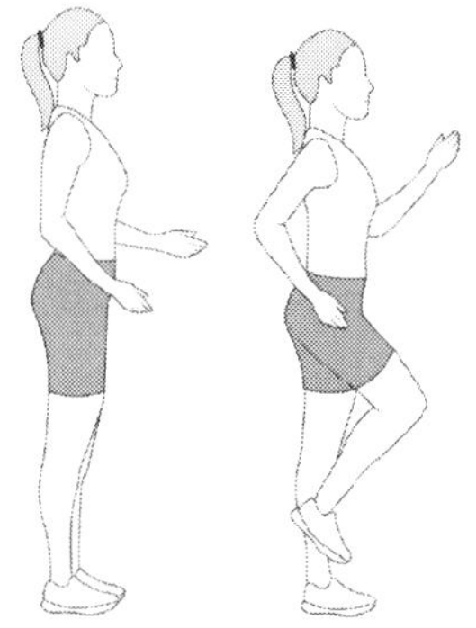

8. Standing Quad Stretch (15-30 secs)

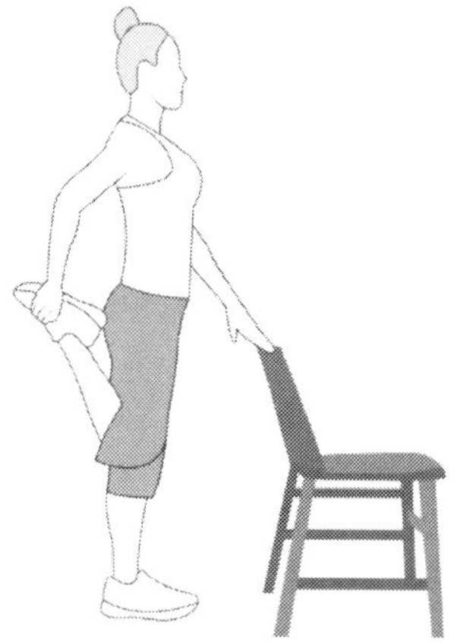

9. Seated Hamstring Stretch (15-30 secs)

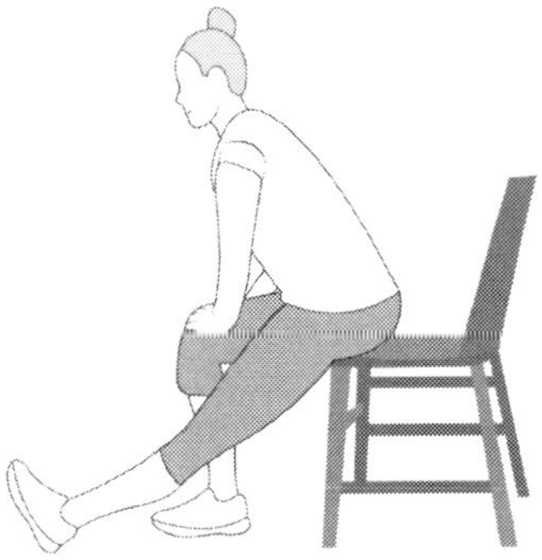

10. Calf Wall Stretch (15-30 secs)

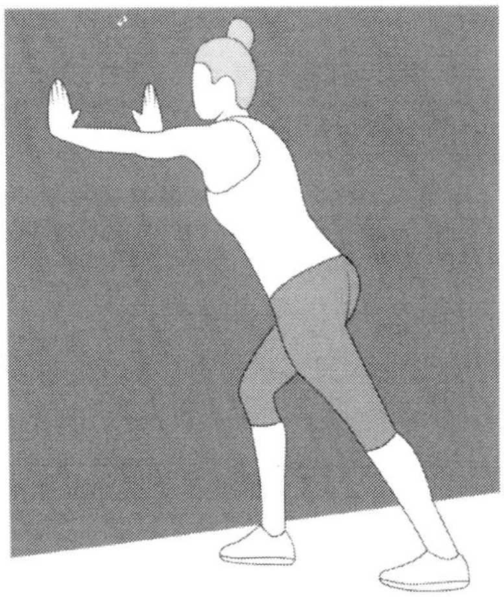

11. Sideways Shuffle (1 min)

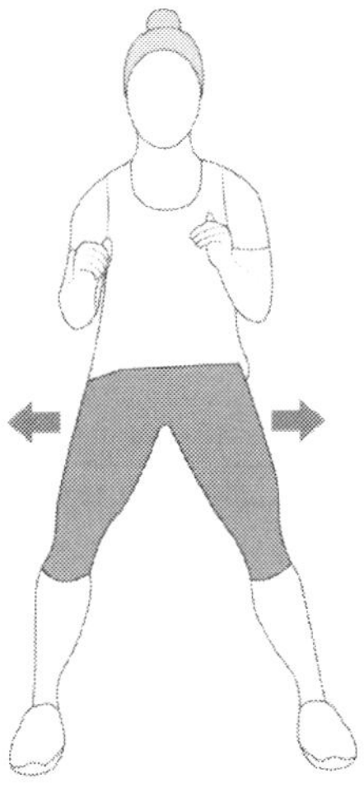

12. Knee Circles (15-30 secs each way)

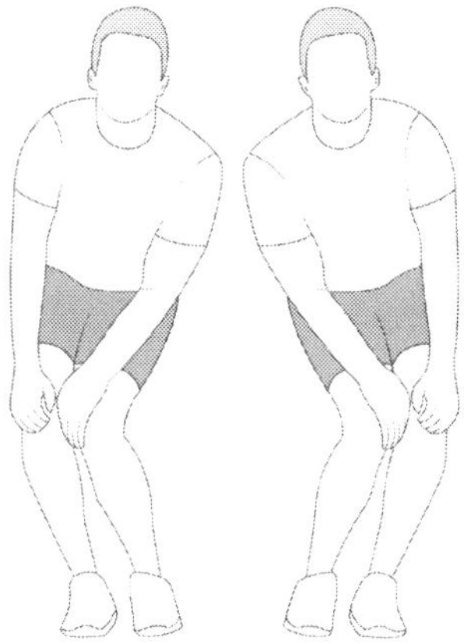

13. Ankle Circles (15-30 secs)

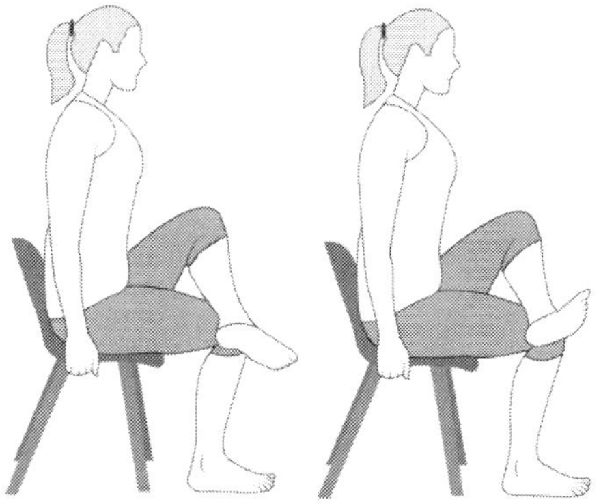

Foundations (Beginner), Full Body Workout

Stretching and Warm-up (5-10 mins)

This workout contains ten of the more basic yet essential exercises from Chapter 8 and is designed to give you a good foundation. The exercises start with the upper body, move to the core, and end with the lower body.

The number of suggested repetitions or times will be listed next to the exercise. Your workout pace should be a comfortable, slow to medium tempo. If using weights is too difficult, do the exercise without dumbbells.

Note: In between each exercise, do a slow March in Place, and Relaxed Arm Shake for approximately 15 seconds. This activity will allow your muscles to recover (important in strength training) and keep your blood flowing into the next exercise.

Total workout time: About 15 minutes

1. The Ostrich Neck (10-12 times)

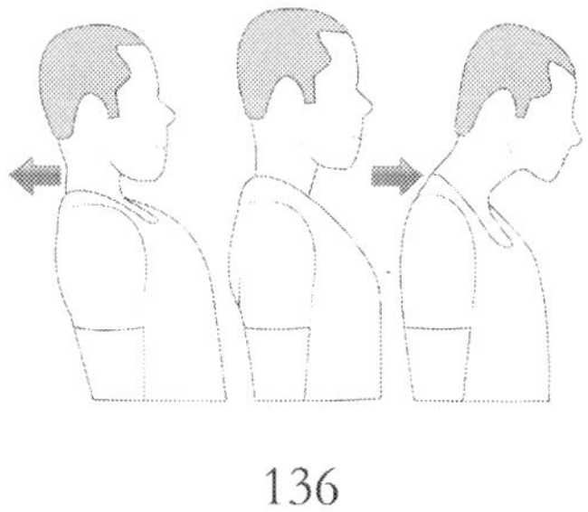

2. Shoulder Squeezes (10-12 times)

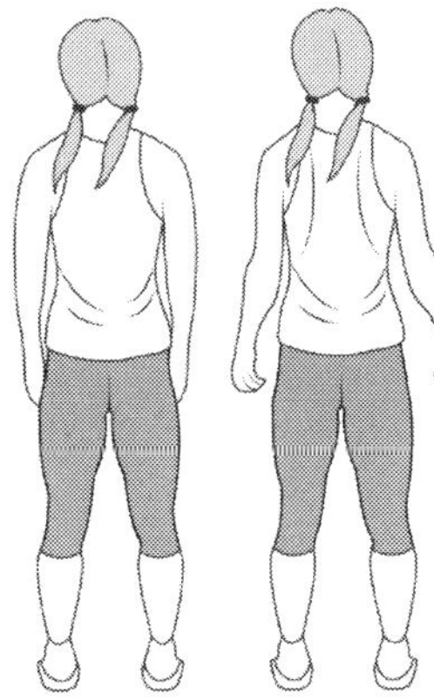

3. Arm Circles (15-20 times each direction)

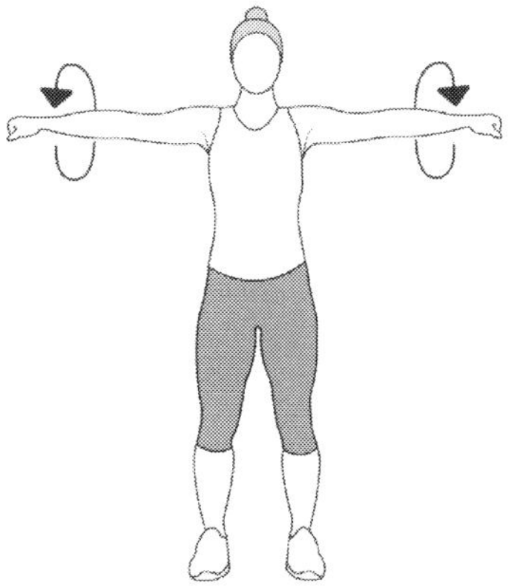

4. Seated Chest Squeezes (12-15 times)

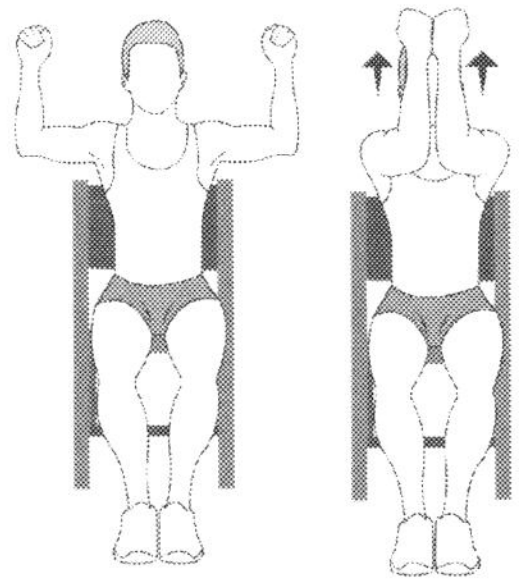

5. Standing Bicep Curls (12-15 per arm)

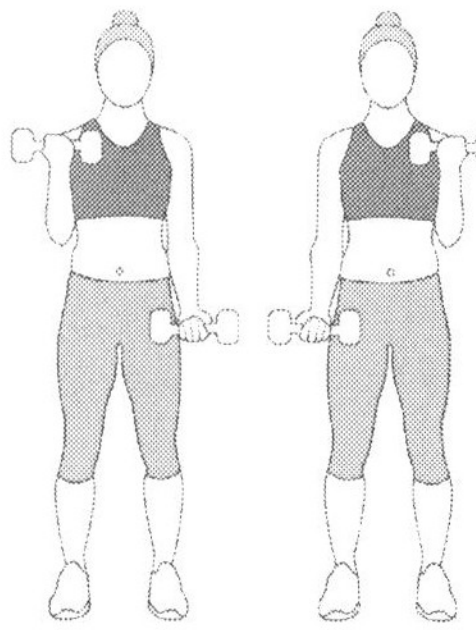

6. Torso Turns (full turn 5 times)

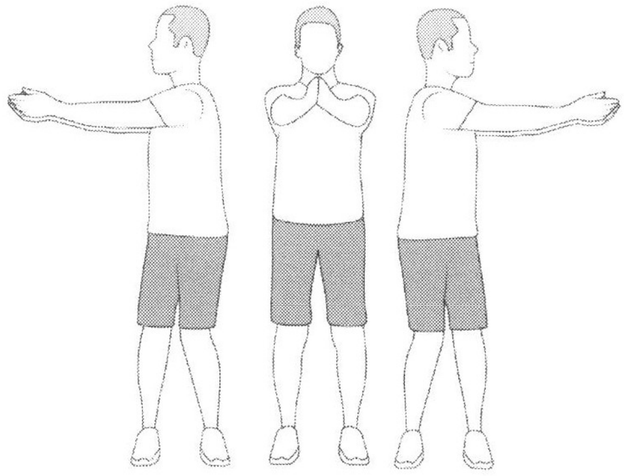

7. Lateral Stepping (10 per leg)

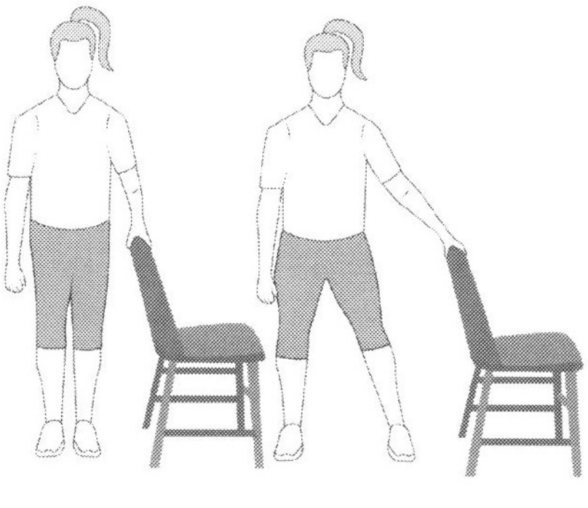

8. The Tightrope (1 minute)

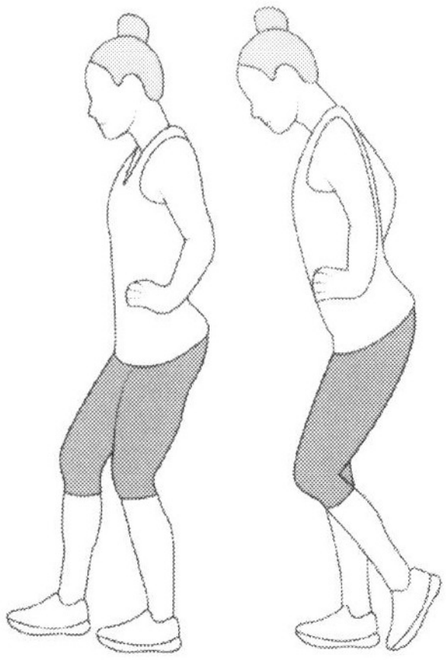

9. Standing Hip Abduction (8-10 per leg)

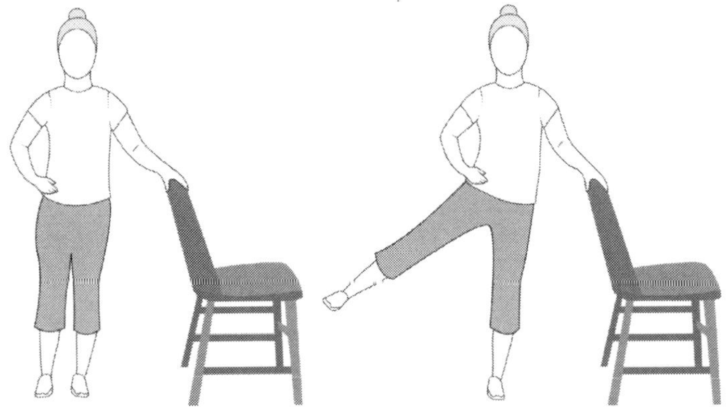

10. Chair Calf Raises (10-12 times)

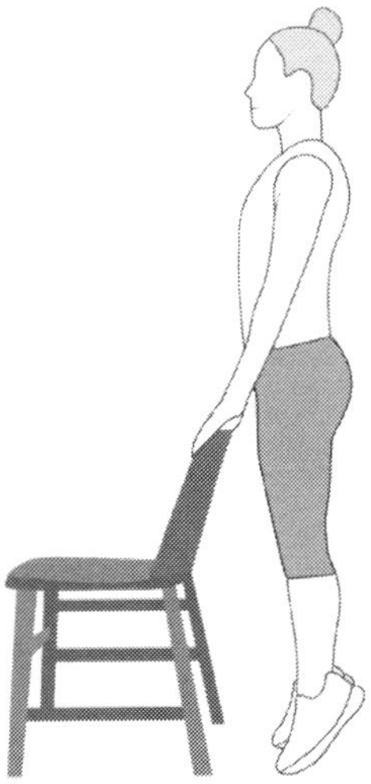

Next Steps (Intermediate), Full Body Workout

Stretching and Warm-up (5-10 mins)

This workout contains ten intermediate-level exercises from Chapter 8 and is designed to provide the next step in your workout routines. The exercises start with the upper body, move to the core, and end with the lower body.

The number of suggested repetitions or times will be listed next to the exercise. Your workout pace should be a comfortable, slow to medium tempo.

Note: In between each exercise, do a slow March in Place, and Relaxed Arm Shake for approximately 15 seconds. This activity will allow your muscles to recover (important in strength training) and keep your blood flowing into the next exercise.

Total workout time: About 15-20 minutes

1. Neck Side Press (10-15 secs per side)

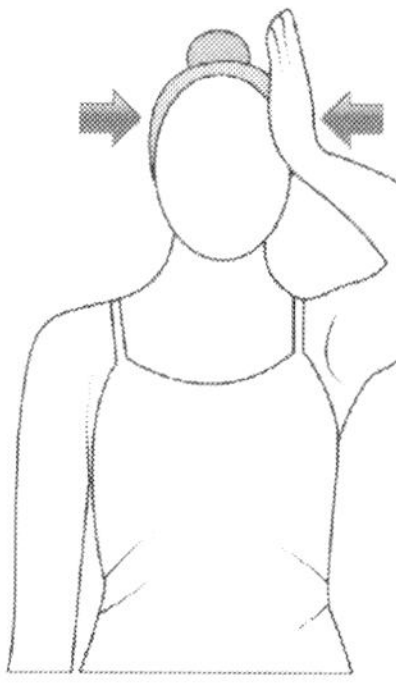

2. Wall Angels (10-12 times)

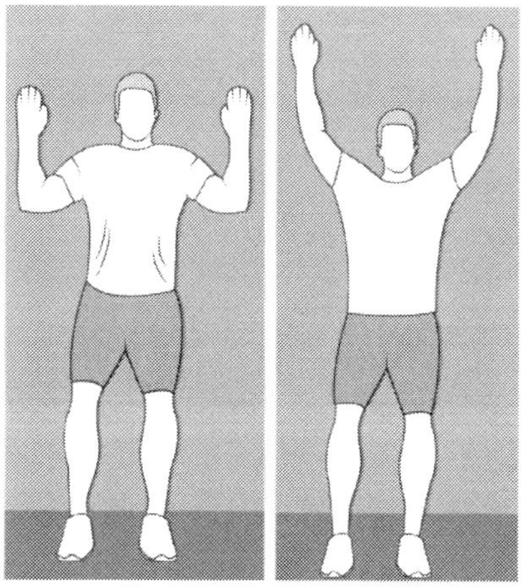

3. Wall Pushups (12-15 times)

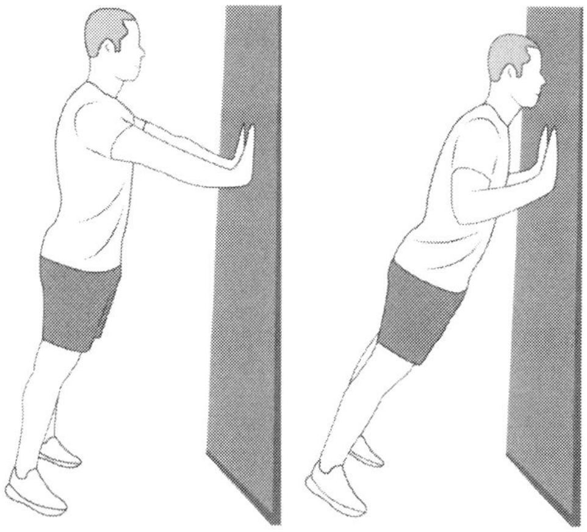

4. Hammer Curls (10-12 times)

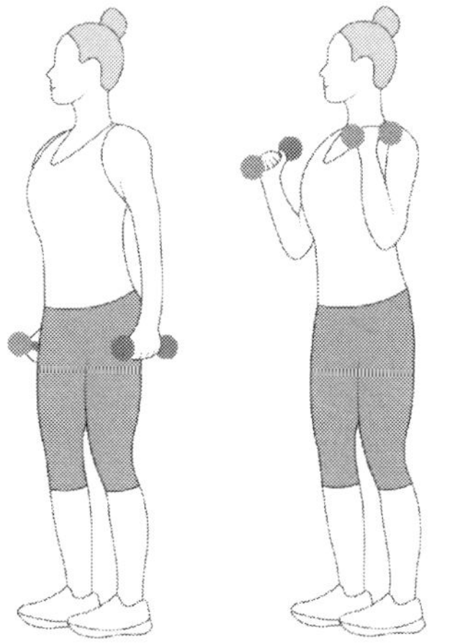

5. Balance Walking (1 minute)

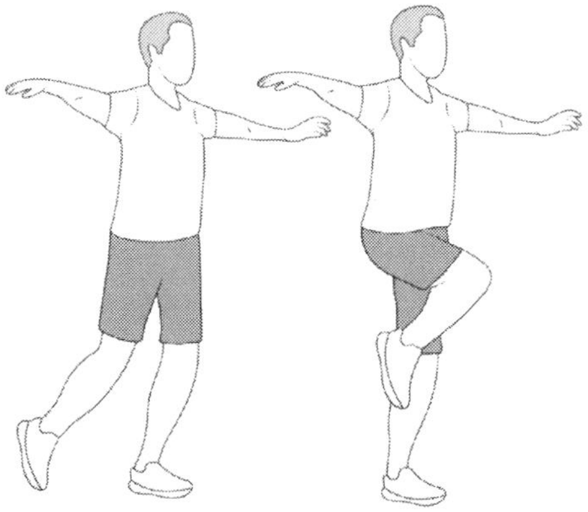

6. Bent Leg Toe Taps (10 per leg)

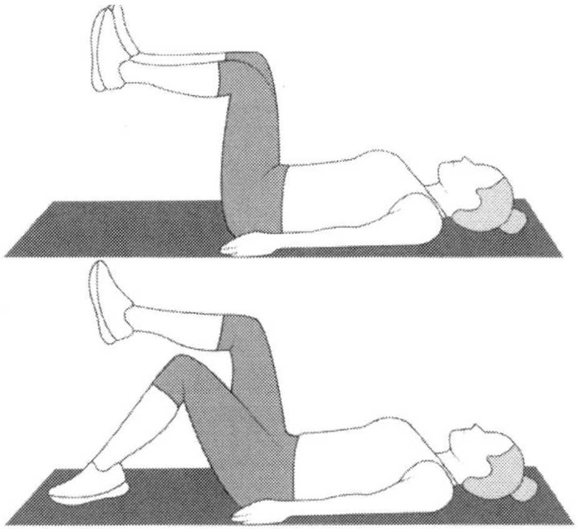

7. Clock Reaches (5 per side)

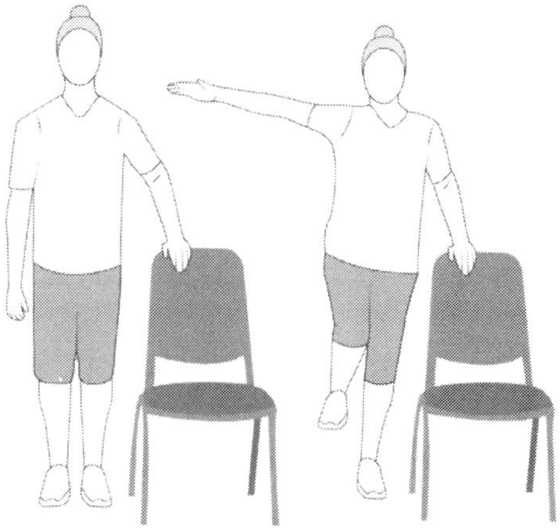

8. Mini Lunges (10 per leg)

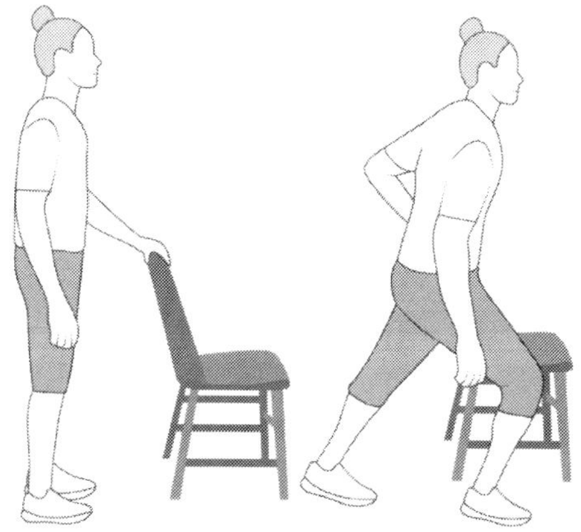

9. Leg Extensions (10-12 per leg)

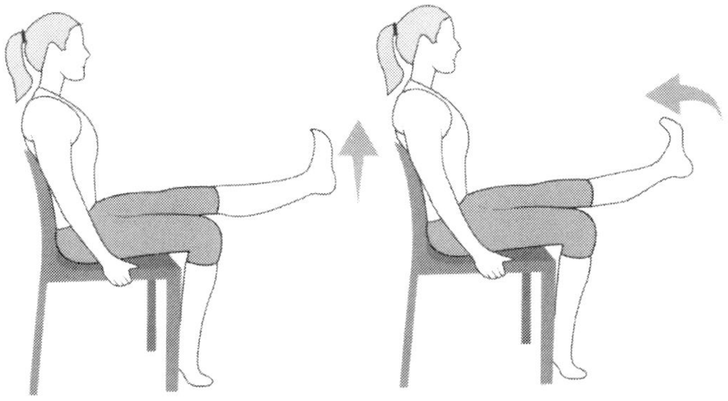

10. Mule Kickbacks (10 times per leg)

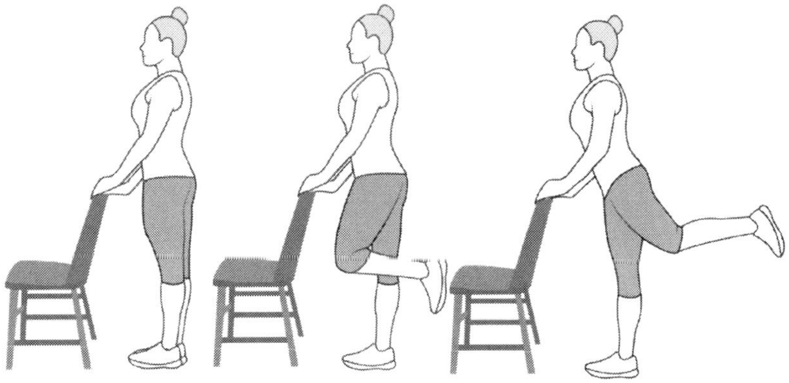

The Tip-Top 10 (Advanced), Full Body Workout

Stretching and Warm-up (5-10 mins)

This workout contains ten intermediate and advanced level exercises from Chapter 8. It is designed as a "point of arrival" workout, and your shape is now becoming "tip-top." The exercises start with the upper body, move to the core, and end with the lower body.

The number of suggested repetitions or times will be listed next to the exercise. Your workout pace should be a comfortable, medium tempo.

Note: In between each exercise, do a slow March in Place, and Relaxed Arm Shake for approximately 15 seconds. This activity will allow your muscles to recover (important in strength training) and keep your blood flowing into the next exercise.

Total workout time: About 20 minutes

1. Car Drivers (8-12 times)

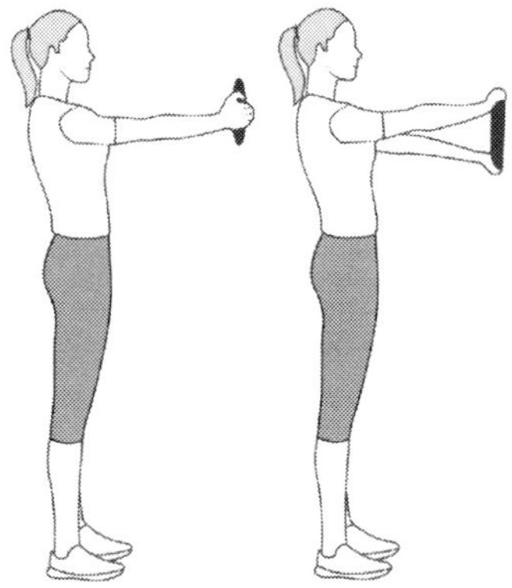

2. Front Shoulder Raises (12-15 per arm)

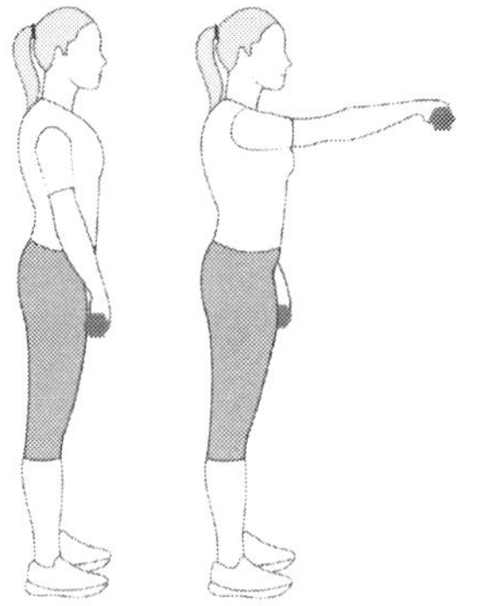

3. Chest Openers (12-15 times)

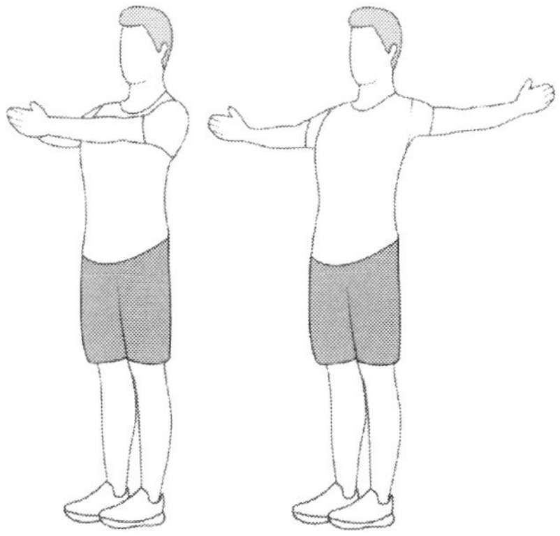

4. Cross Chest Curls (12-15 times)

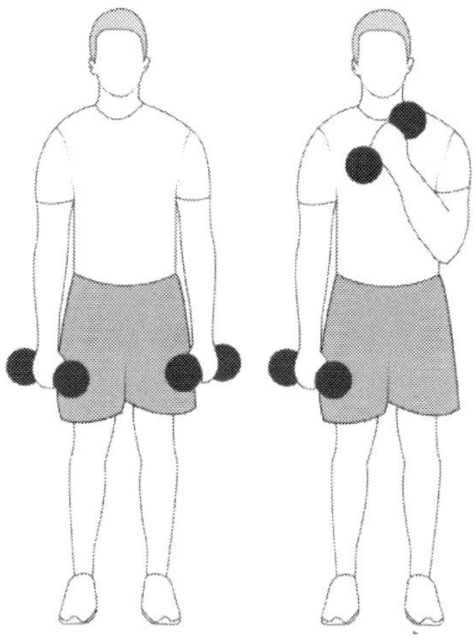

5. The Tightrope (2 minutes)

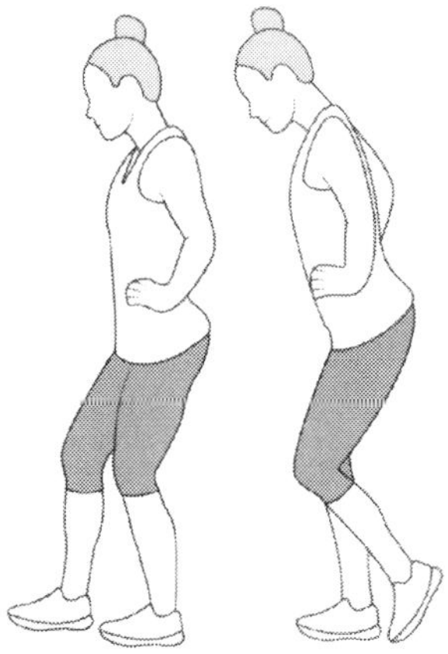

6. Mountain Climbers (12-15 times)

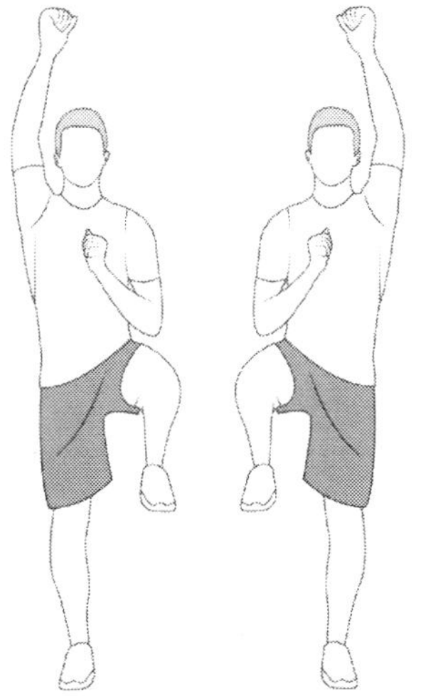

7. Hip Hinges (10-12 times)

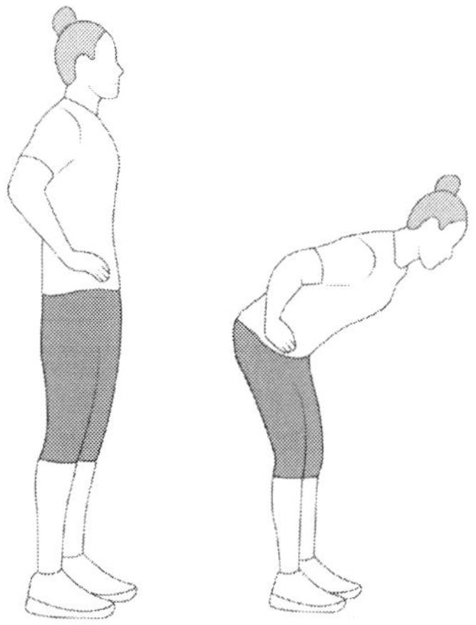

8. Side Lunges (10 per leg)

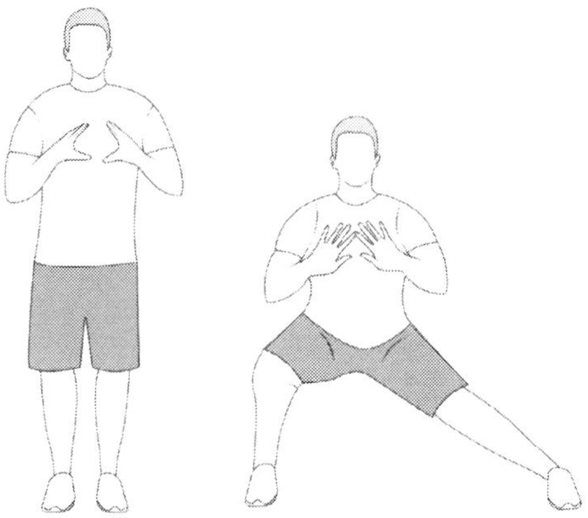

9. Chair Squats (10-12 times)

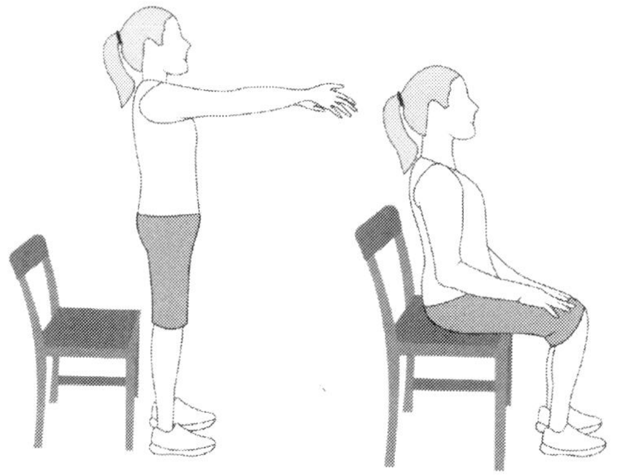

10. Weighted Calf Raises (10-12 times)

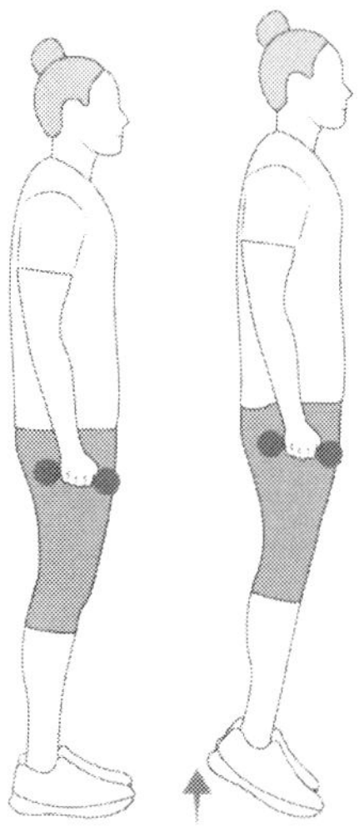

Balance 5, Core Workout

Stretching and Warm-up (5-10 mins)

This workout contains five foundational core exercises from Chapter 8 and focuses on improving balance and coordination.

In this workout, do each exercise only once. However, once you have mastered it, you can run through it again at your comfort level. You can also replace any core exercise with any on the list in Ch. 8 based on your comfort level and pain tolerance for that exercise.

The number of suggested repetitions or times will be listed next to the exercise. Your workout pace should be a comfortable, slow to medium tempo.

Note: In between each exercise, do a slow March in Place for approximately 10-15 seconds. This activity will allow your muscles to rest and keep your blood flowing into the next exercise. Remember that good form is vital.

Total workout time: About 10-15 minutes

1. Lateral Stepping (10 times per leg)

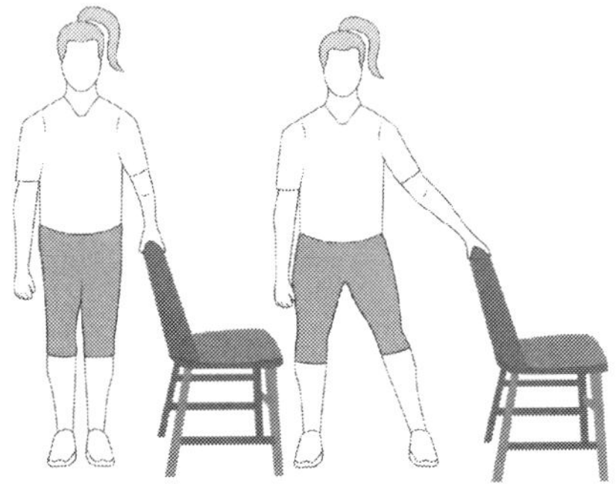

2. Dead Bugs (10-12 times)

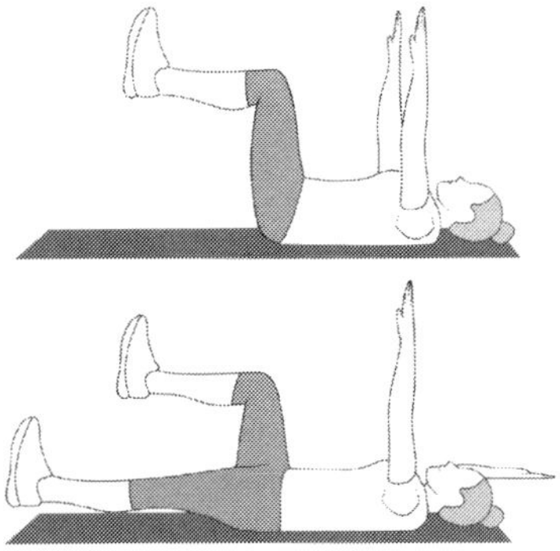

3. Mountain Climbers (12-15 times)

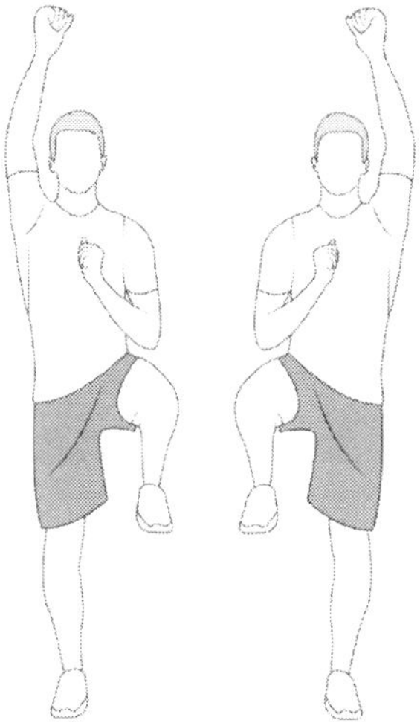

4. Knee to Chest (10 per leg)

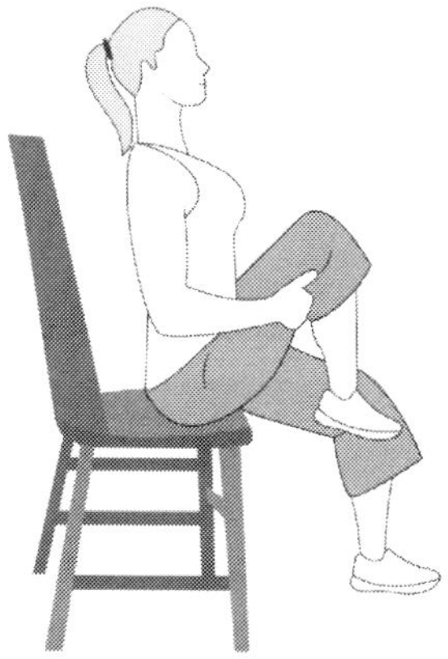

5. Clock Reaches (5 per side)

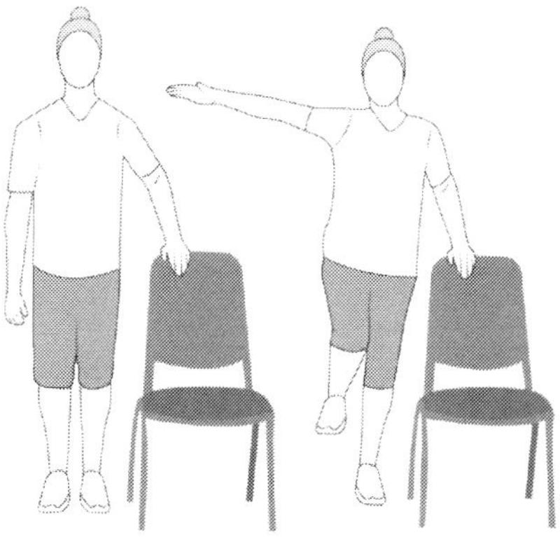

Balance 7, Core Workout

Stretching and Warm-up (5-10 mins)

This workout contains seven intermediate core exercises from Chapter 8 and focuses on improving balance and coordination.

In this workout, do each exercise only once. However, once you have mastered it, you can run through it again at your comfort level. You can also replace any core exercise with any on the list in Chapter 8 based on your comfort level and pain tolerance for that exercise.

The number of suggested repetitions or times will be listed next to the exercise. Your workout pace should be a comfortable, slow to medium tempo.

Note: In between each exercise, do a slow March in Place for approximately 10-15 seconds. This activity will allow your muscles to rest and keep your blood flowing into the next exercise. Remember that good form is vital.

Total workout time: About 15-20 minutes

1. The Flamingo (12-15 times)

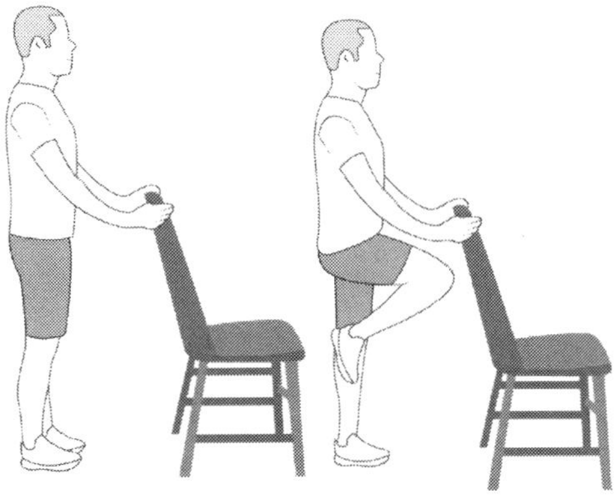

2. Abdominal Bridges (10-12 times)

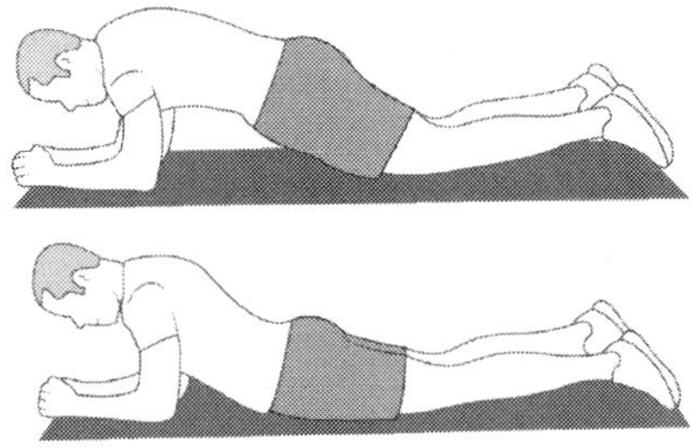

3. Knees to Chest (10-12 times)

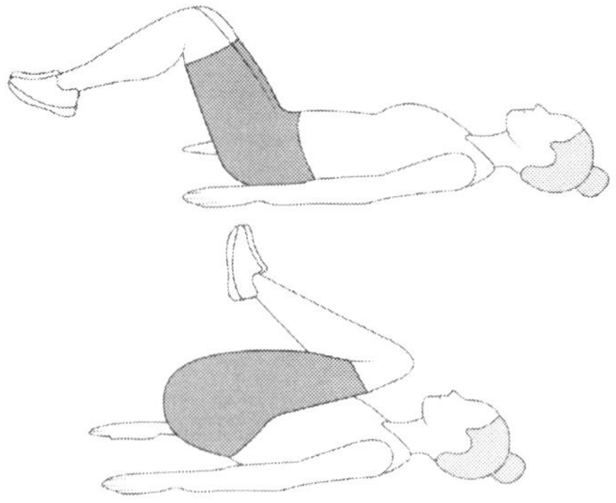

4. Pelvic Tilts (10-12 times)

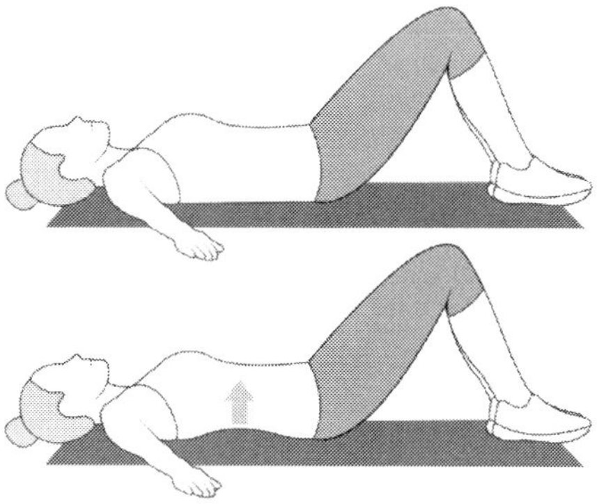

5. Glute Bridges (10-12 times)

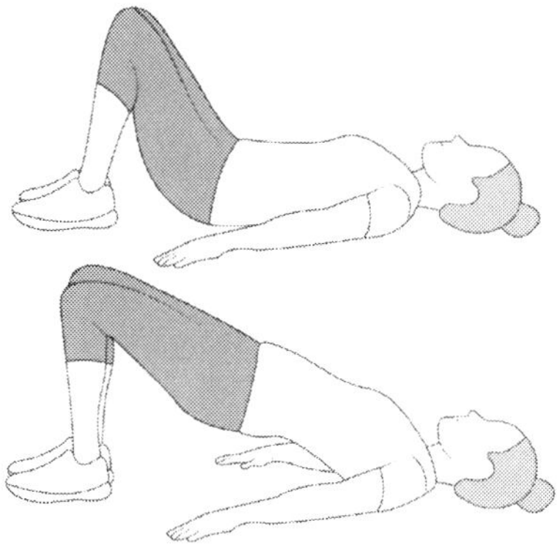

6. Clock Reaches (5 times per side)

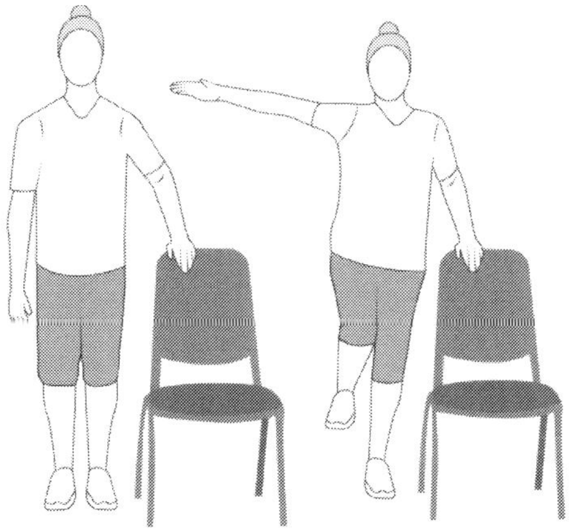

7. Step Ups (10-15 times)

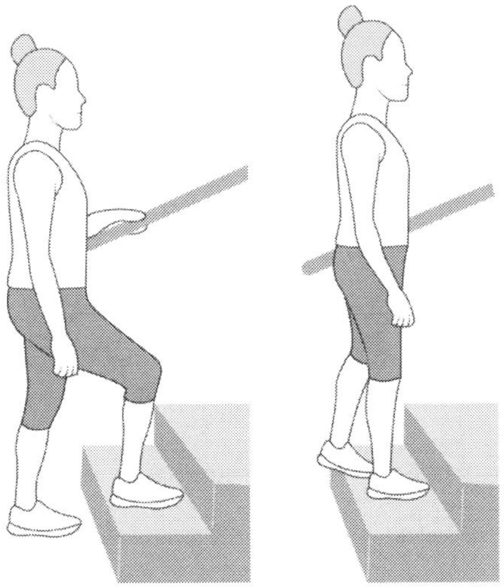

Quickie Cardio, Mini Full Body Workout

Stretching (5 mins)

This workout contains seven exercises from Chapter 8 and focuses on efficient training and cardiovascular health.

In this workout, do each exercise only once unless indicated. You can replace any similar exercise with any on the list in Chapter 8 based on your comfort level and pain tolerance for the exercise. The number of suggested repetitions or times will be listed next to the exercise. Your workout pace should be a medium-fast tempo. Because this is designed to keep your heart rate up, not much rest is needed between exercises.

Total workout time: About 10-15 minutes

1. Marching in Place (30 seconds)

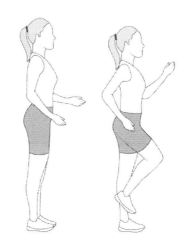

2. Arm Swings (12-15 times)

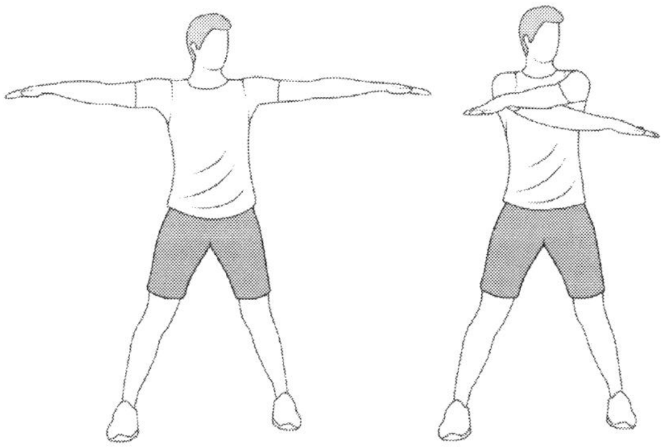

3. Dead Bugs (12-15 times)

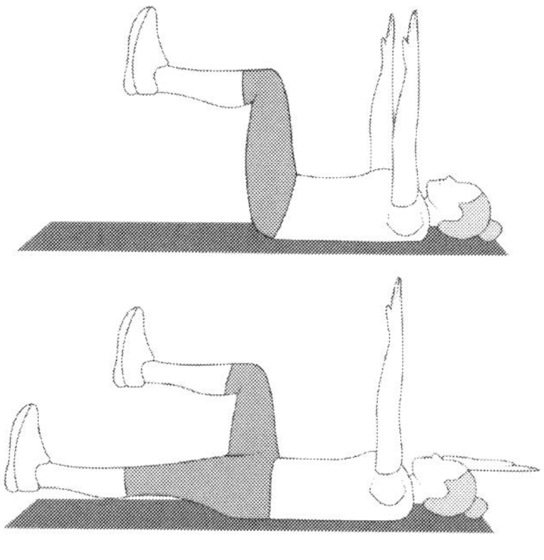

4. Sideways Shuffle (30 seconds)

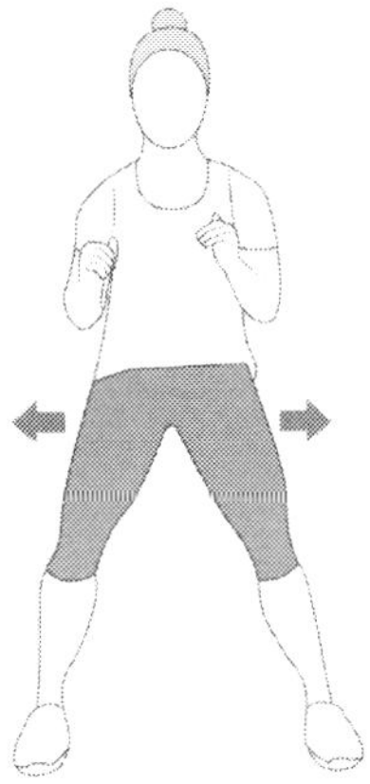

5. Chest Openers (15 times)

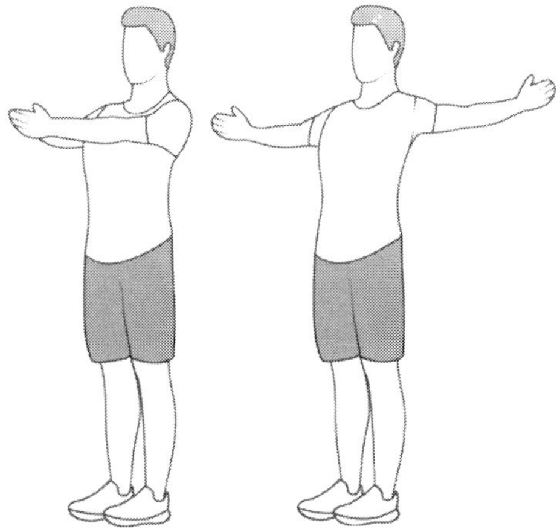

6. Mountain Climbers (12-15 times)

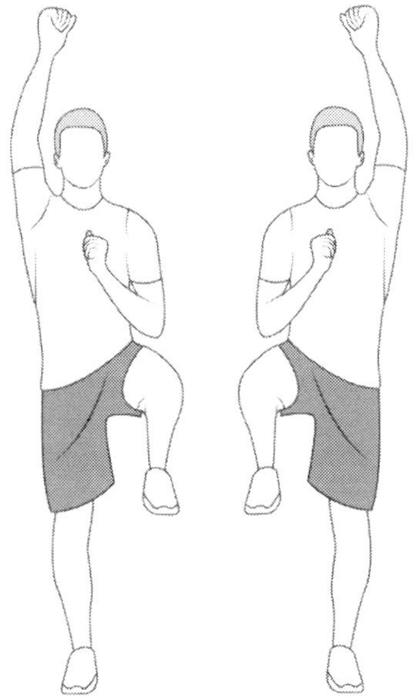

7. Fighter Squats (15-20 times)

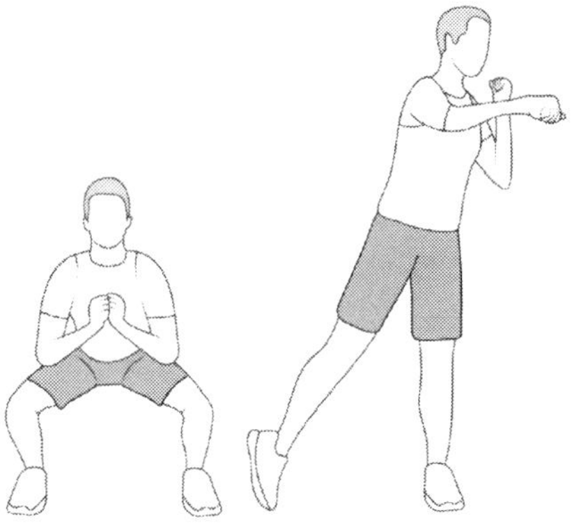

8. Marching in Place (30 seconds)

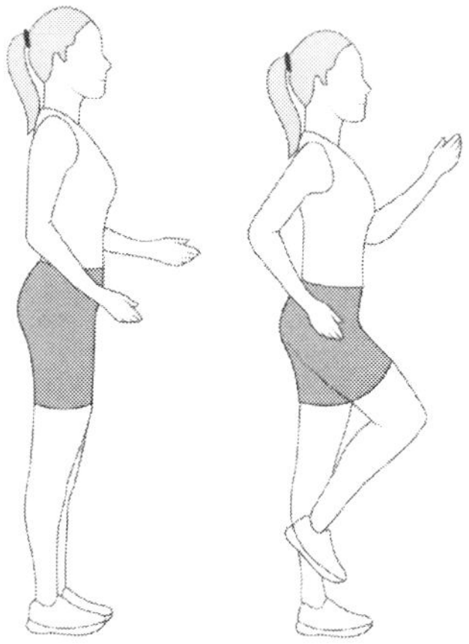

Pain Relief Workouts

Stretching and Warm-up (5-10 mins)

The following workouts contain exercises and stretch from Chapter 8 that will help various pain points.

In these workouts, do each exercise only once. You can replace any similar stretching exercise with any on the list in Chapter 8 based on your comfort level and pain tolerance.

Do each exercise slowly 10-15 times unless otherwise indicated. Remember that good form is critical. If you are feeling any significant pain, stop the exercise, try to stretch the body part gently, and move on to another exercise. Slight muscle discomfort is a normal part of strength training, but we do not want to injure ourselves. Because these are primarily stretching exercises, rest only needs to be about 10-15 seconds between exercises.

Total workout time: About 15 minutes each workout

Pain Workout 1: Neck, Back, Shoulders

1. Rolling Neck (12-15 times)

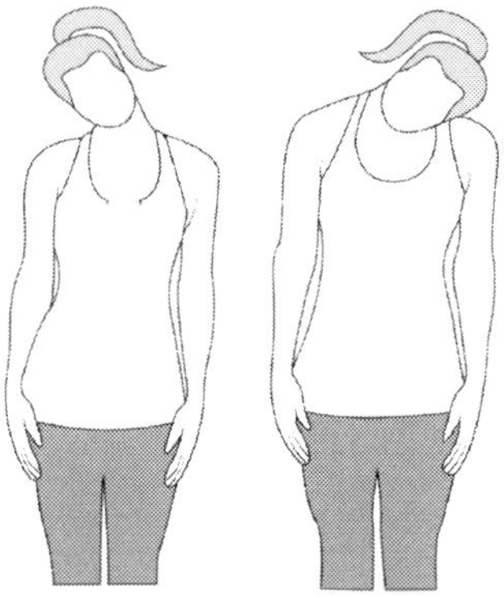

2. The Ostrich (12-15 times)

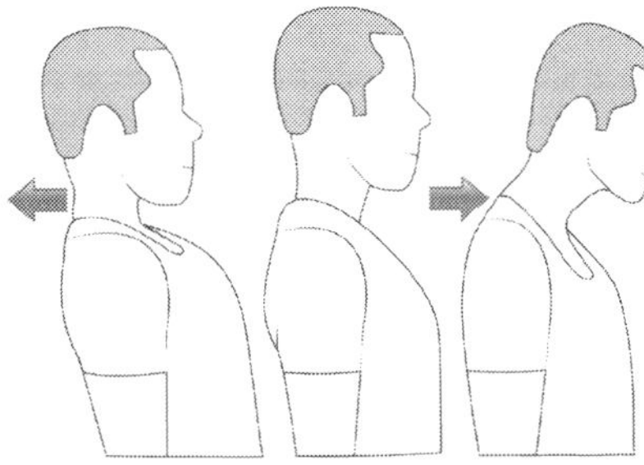

3. Prayer Stretches (8-10 times)

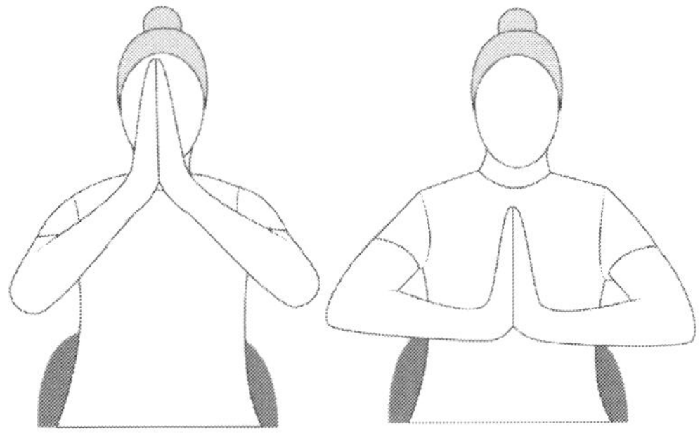

4. Arm Swings (30 seconds)

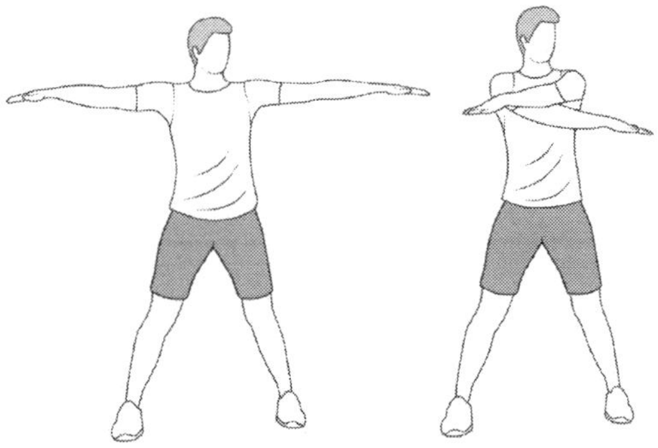

5. Shoulder Pulls (10 times)

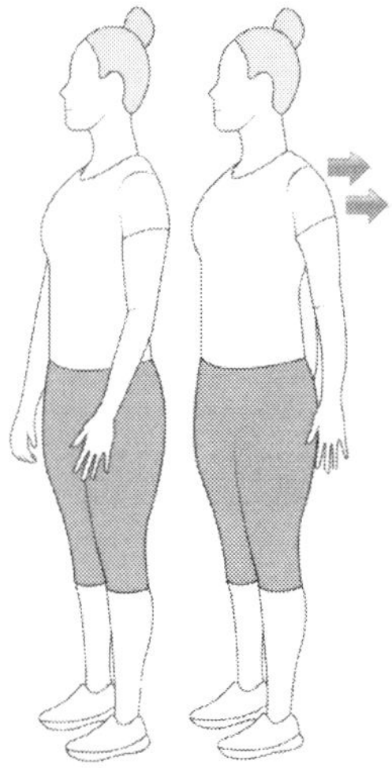

6. One Arm Hugs (5 times per arm)

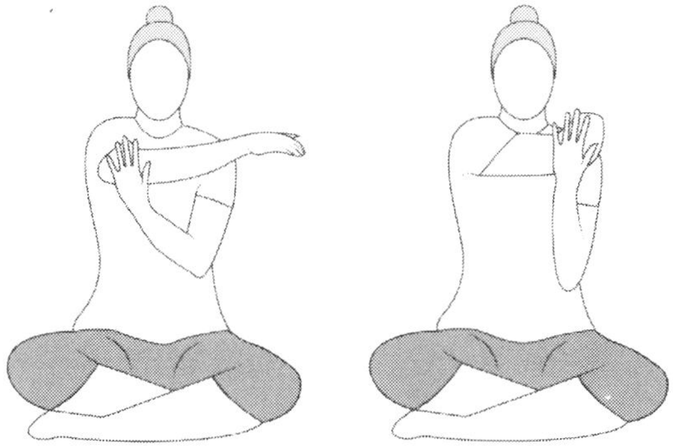

7. Wall Angels (10 times)

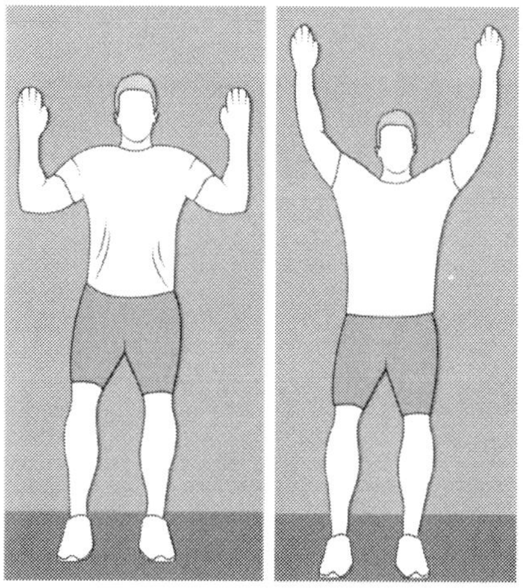

Pain Workout 2: Hips, Knees, and Ankles

1. Hip Swings (10 per leg)

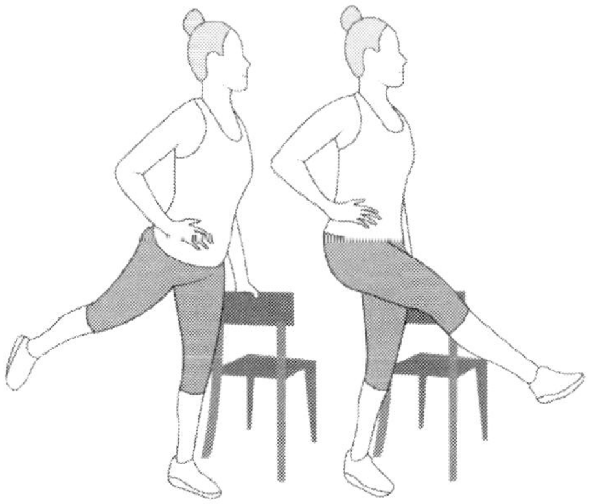

2. Hip Circles (10 times each way)

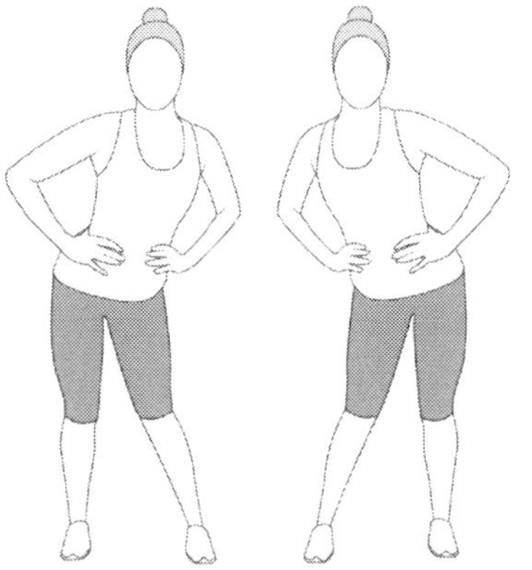

3. Calf Wall Stretch (5 per leg)

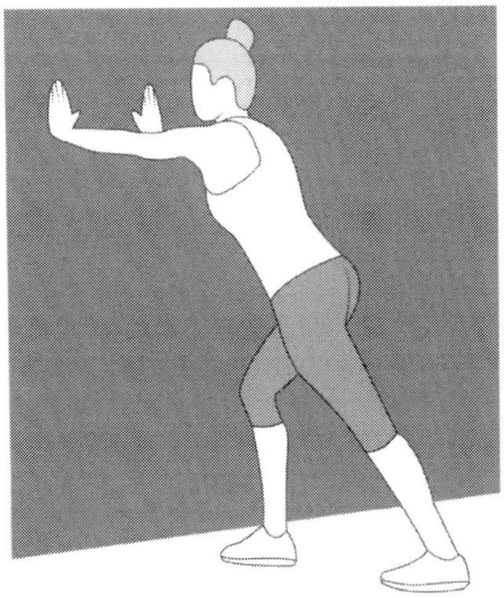

4. Marching in Place (30 seconds)

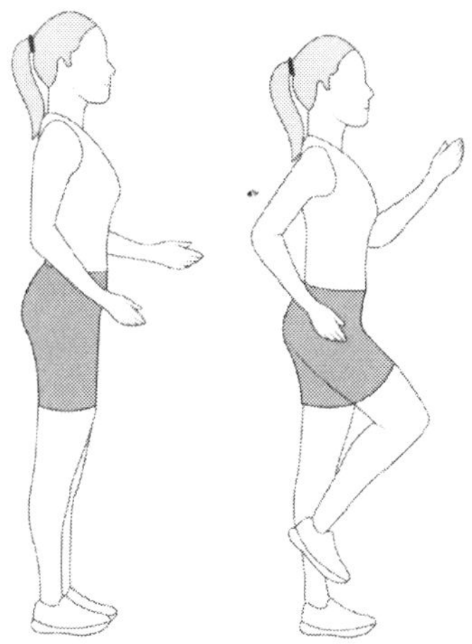

5. Knee Circles (5 times per way)

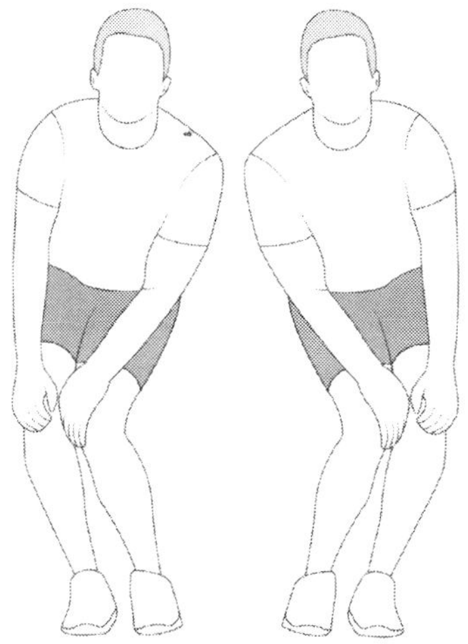

6. Leg Extensions (10 per leg)

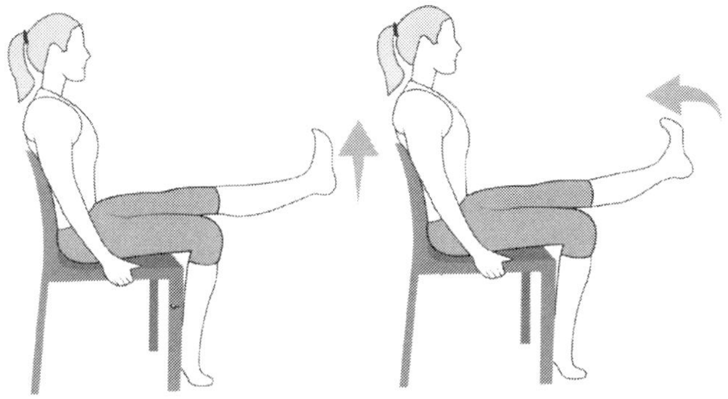

7. Ankle Circles (10 per leg)

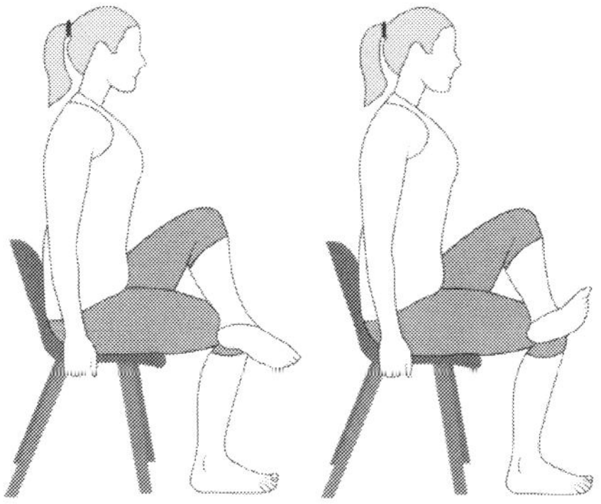

Pain Workout 3: Sciatica, Back

1. Smooth Twists (30 secs)

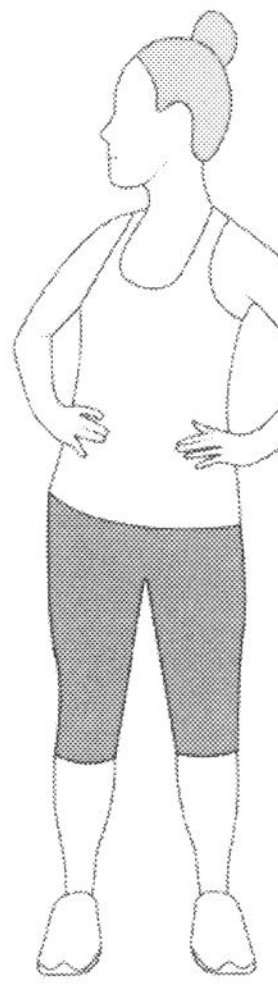

2. Overhead Side Stretch (5 per side)

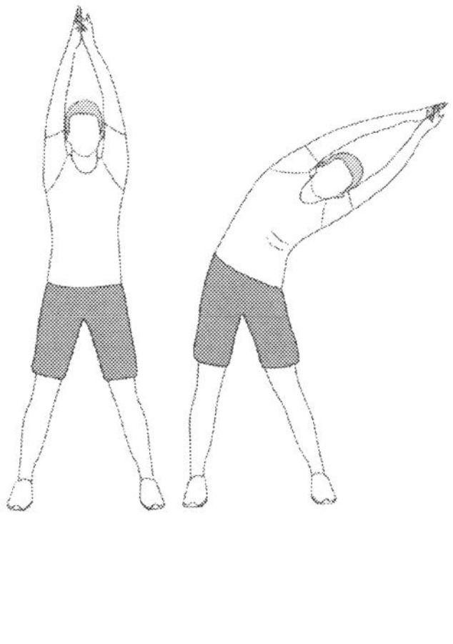

3. Mountain Climbers (30 secs slow)

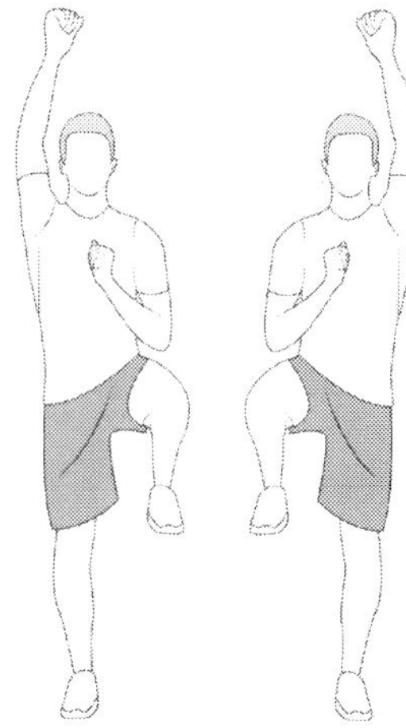

4. Cat-Cows (8-10 times)

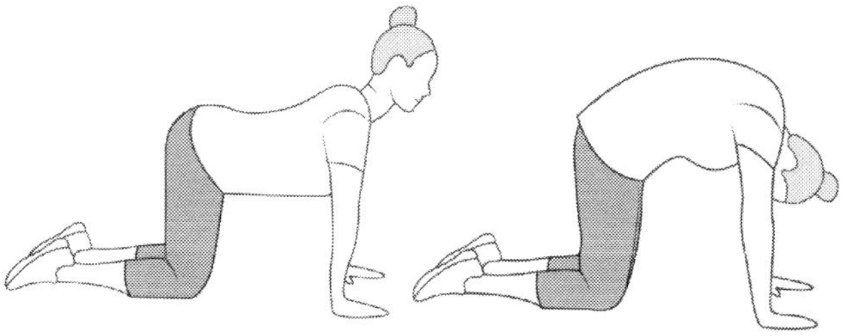

5. Glute Bridges (8-10 times)

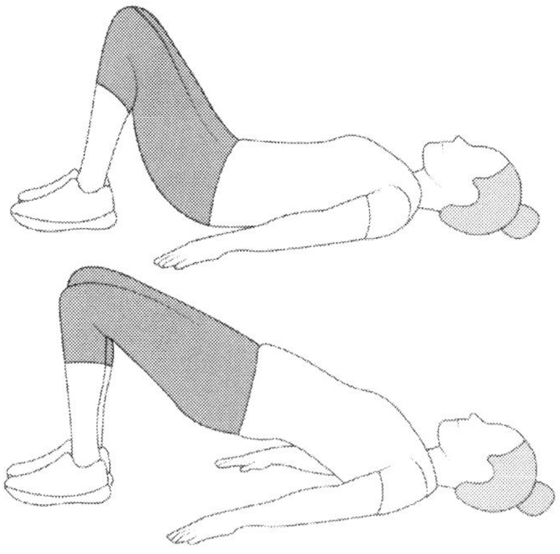

6. Knees to Chest (10 times)

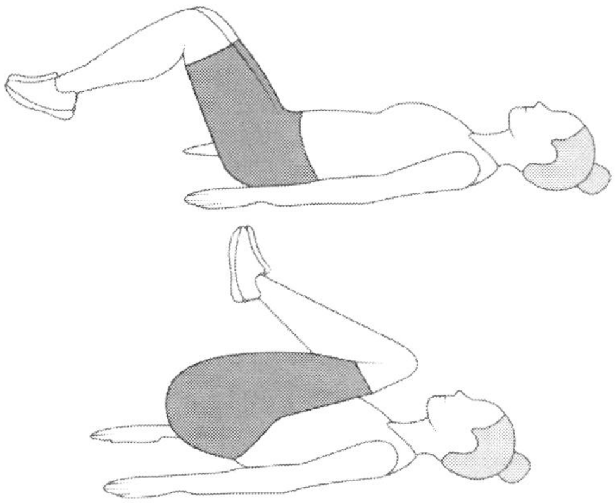

7. Child's Pose (8-10 times)

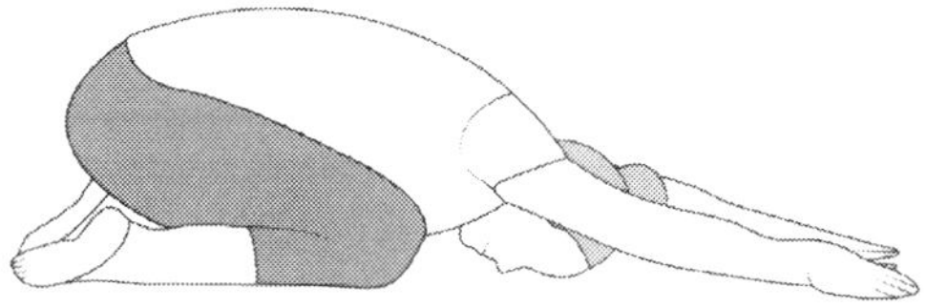

Pain Workout 4: Wrist and Elbows

Note: Try this workout without weights first. If you feel strong enough, slowly work the weights into the routine.

1. Wrist Stretches (60 secs per wrist)

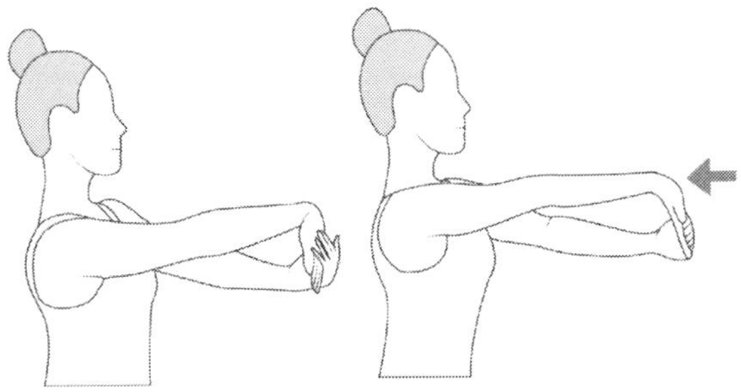

2. Wrist Curl Flexion (10 times)

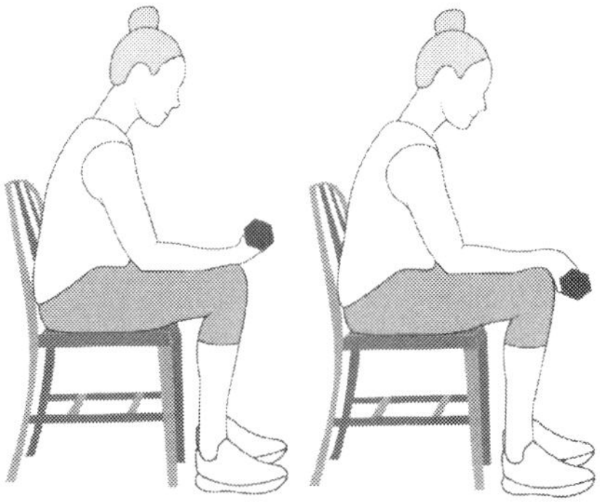

3. Wrist Curl Extensions (10 times)

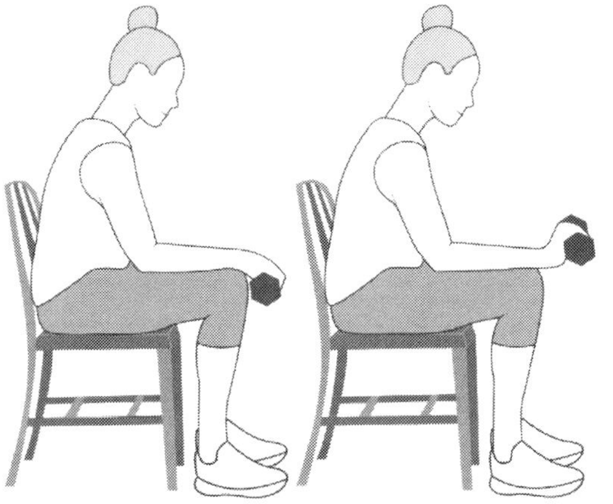

4. Relaxed Arm Shakeouts (15-20 secs)

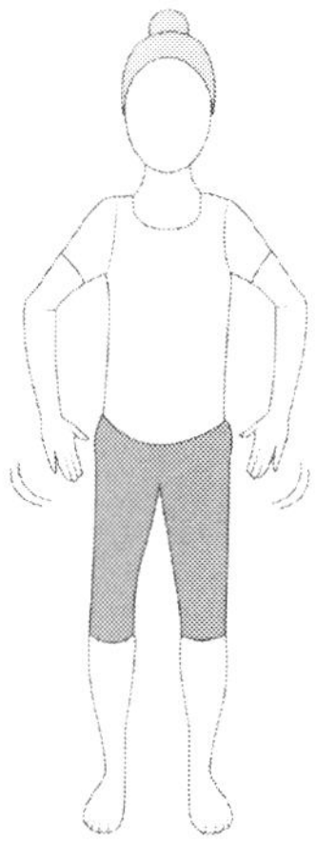

5. Prayer Stretches (10 times)

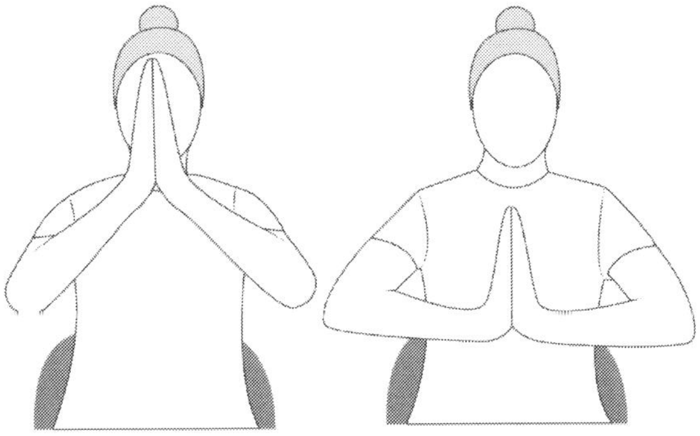

6. Bicep Curls (10 times per arm)

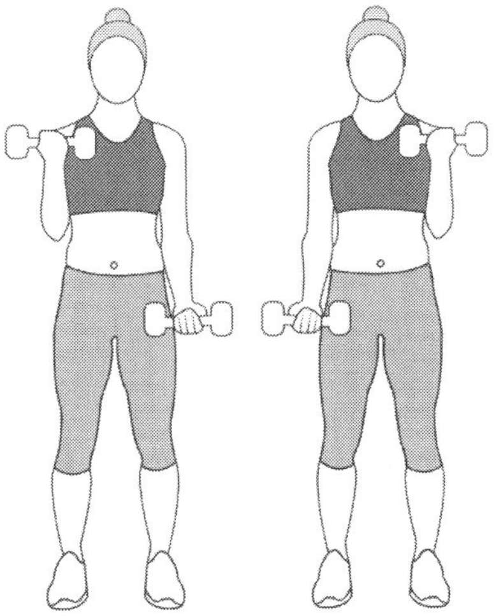

7. Bicep Stretches (5-7 times)

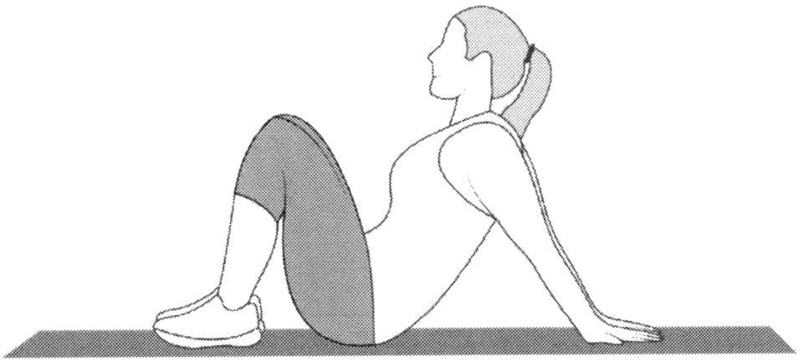

Give Me Strength Special, Full Body Workout

Stretching and Warm-up (5-10 mins)

This workout contains 11 intermediate to advanced level exercises from Chapter 8 and is designed as an advanced, next-level routine. The exercises start with the upper body, move to the core, and end with the lower body.

In this workout, do each exercise only once. Based on your comfort level and pain tolerance, you can replace any exercise with any on the list in Chapter 8 (per category).

The number of suggested repetitions or times will be listed next to the exercise. Your workout pace should be medium tempo.

Note: In between each exercise, do a slow March in Place, and Relaxed Arm Shake for approximately 15 seconds. This activity will allow your muscles to recover (important in strength training) and keep your blood flowing into the next exercise.

Total workout time: About 25-30 minutes

1. Side Shoulder Raises (12-15 times)

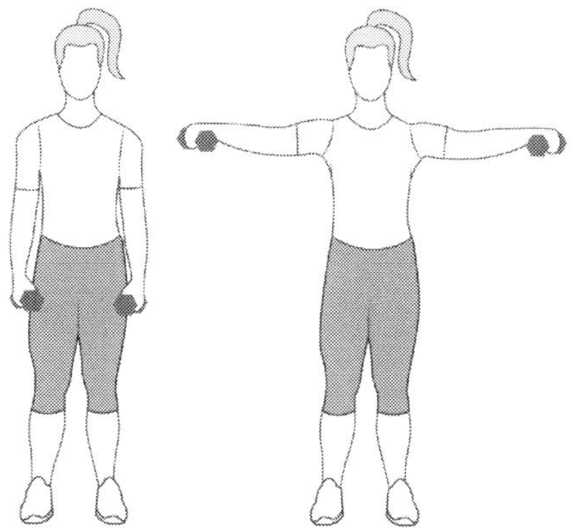

2. Bent Over Rows (10 per arm)

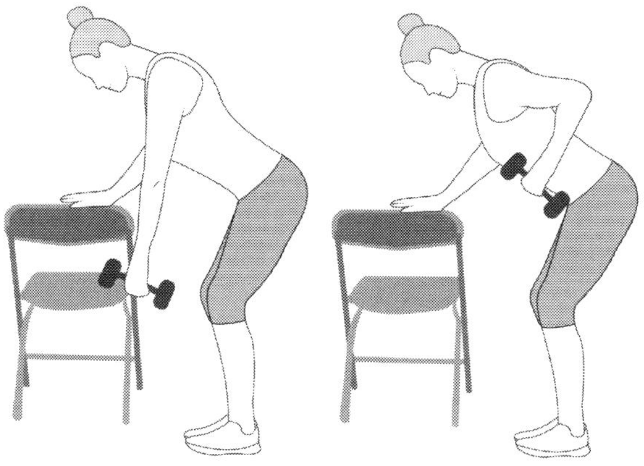

3. Tricep Extensions (12-15 times)

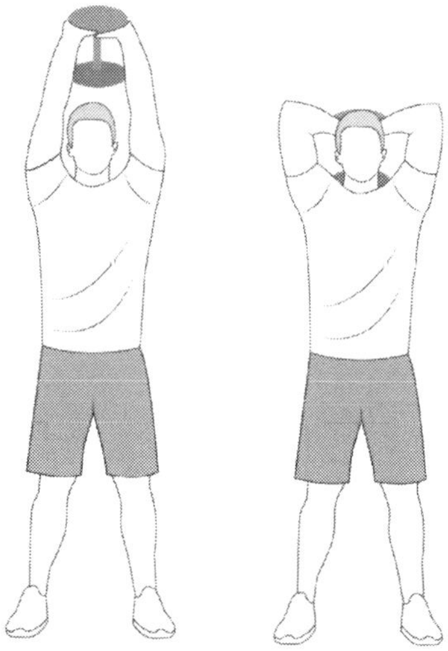

4. Seated Dips (12-15 times)

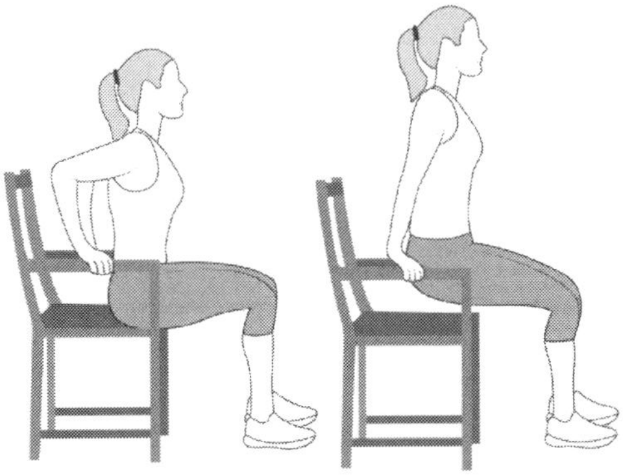

5. Abdominal Bridges (10 times)

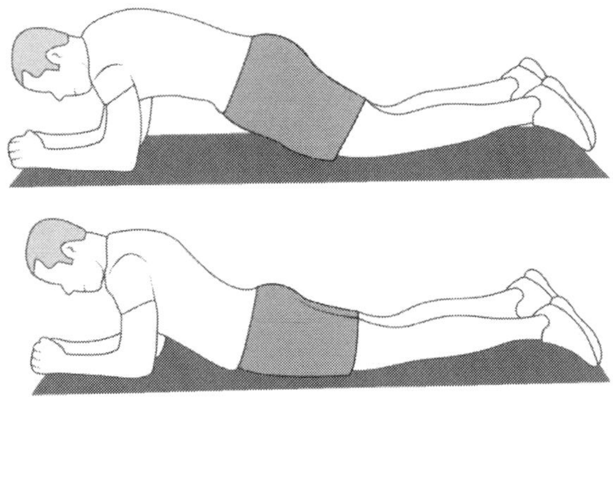

6. Dead Bugs (10-15 times)

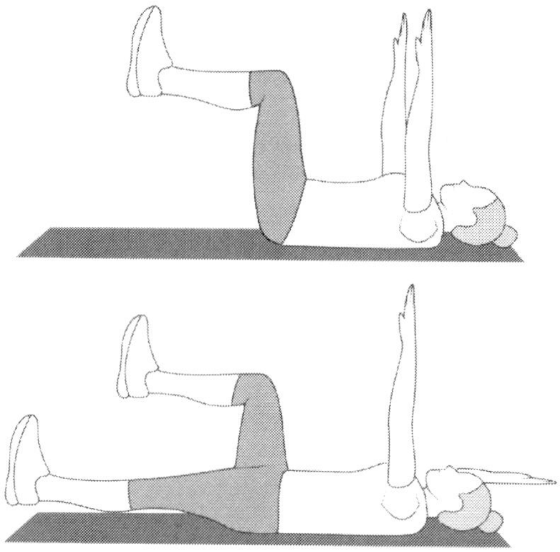

7. The Superman (10-15 times)

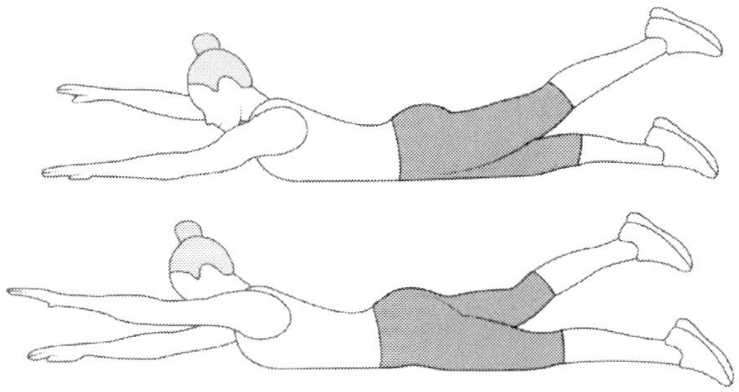

8. Hamstring Mule Kickbacks (10 per leg)

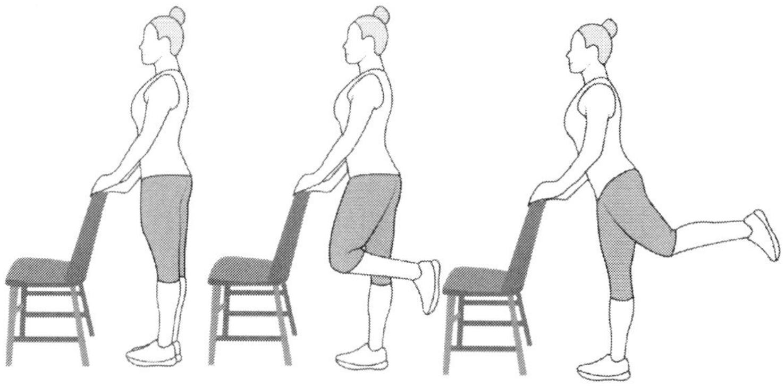

9. Single Leg Forward Reach (5 per leg)

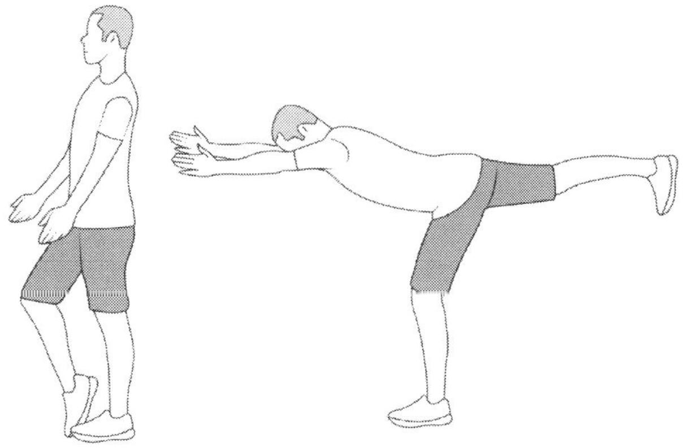

10. Squatting Reaches (10 times)

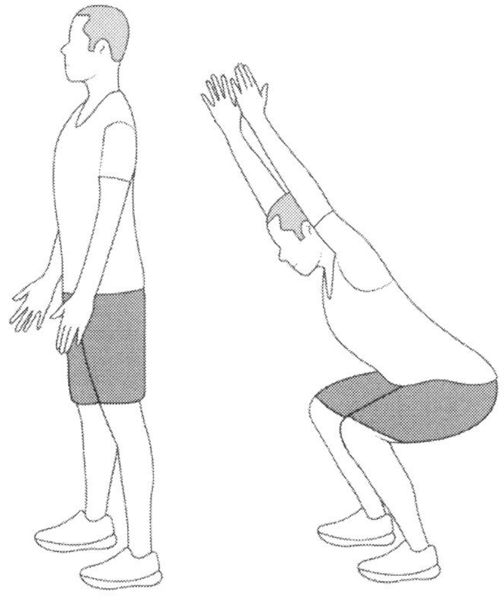

11. Lunging Bicep Curls (5-7 per leg)

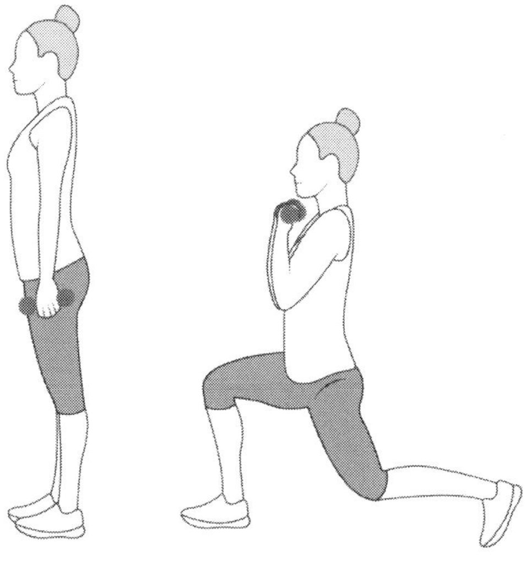

Conclusion

In these nine chapters, we have covered a lot of information, from understanding the excellent benefits of strength and conditioning training, to creating an individual plan, to discovering the multitudinous exercise options that now lay at your fingertips.

Believe it or not, when you first picked up this book, you took a big step by just acknowledging you need a good solution for better health. Having this kind of self-awareness and finally doing something about it is half the battle. So please do not discount how significant of a step that is.

By reading the pages in this book, you have now also succeeded in taking another leap toward accomplishing this mission. Your knowledge of strength and conditioning has grown significantly, as have ideas for practical and strategic ways to use this knowledge.

If you will or are about to apply the principles and exercise directions within these pages, you have also succeeded in making a third leap toward giving yourself a much better opportunity at a better life filled with healthier and happier days.

Despite how comprehensive this book is, there is still a lot we could not cover. Therefore, I highly encourage you to continue to learn all you can. Google, read articles, blogs, more books, etc. And please join our email list and Facebook group (Give Me Strength - Fitness for Seniors) to receive the most current strength and conditioning updates, including excellent nutrition guidance, new exercises and techniques, and tips on goal setting and motivation.

Thank you for joining me on this journey on these pages. The process of researching, outlining, editing, and publishing all the data has been a fantastic adventure for me. I genuinely hope you enjoyed reading it and will keep learning and applying all you know. Please be sure to share with others and help them in the process of feeling better as they age, so you can be there when they cry out for help and say, "Give Me Strength!"

Thank you!

Leave a Quick Review

I would be incredibly grateful if you would please take 60 seconds to write a brief review on Amazon, even if it's just a few sentences.

Visit this webpage to leave a quick Amazon review: www.givemestrengthfitness.com/review or scan this QR code:

Join our Facebook group! Just visit this webpage or scan the QR code below!

http://www.facebook.com/groups/givemestrength

Bibliography

Introduction

- Drash, Wayne. (2019, January 11). *Not Exercising Worse for Your Health Than Smoking, Diabetes and Heart Diseases, Study Reveals.* CNN Health. Retrieved from https://www.cnn.com/2018/10/19/health/study-not-exercising-worse-than-smoking/index.html

Chapter 1

- Hester, S. H. (2015, February 16). *What Happens When We Age and Can We Slow the Aging Process?* The Source. Retrieved from https://www.nuskin.com/content/corpcom/en_US/thesource/healthandfitness/what-happens-when-we-age-and-can-we-slow-the-aging-process-.html
- National Library of Medicine. (n.d.). *Aging Changes in Organs, Tissues and Cells.* Medline Plus. Retrieved fromhttps://medlineplus.gov/ency/article/004012.htm
- Mayo Clinic. (n.d.). *Aging: What to Expect.* Mayo Clinic. Org. Retrieved from https://www.mayoclinic.org/healthy-lifestyle/healthy-aging/in-depth/aging/art-20046070
- Wikipedia. (2022, February 5). *Collagen Loss.* Retrieved fromhttps://en.wikipedia.org/wiki/Collagen_loss
- Penn State Milton S. Hershey Medical Center. (n.d.). *Strength Training Helps Older Adults Live Longer.* Science Daily. Retrieved from https://www.sciencedaily.com/releases/2016/04/160420090406.htm
- Chaplin, B. C. (2019, August 30). *What is Strength and Conditioning?* Strength and Conditioning Education. Retrieved from https://strengthandconditioningeducation.com/what-is-strength-conditioning/
- Trifocus Fitness Academy. (n.d.). *What Exactly is Strength and Conditioning.* Retrieved May 21, 2022, from https://trifocusfitnessacademy.co.za/blog/what-exactly-is-strength-and-conditioning-training/
- Harvard Medical School. (n.d.). *Exercise and aging: Can you walk away from Father Time.* Harvard Health Publishing. Retrieved from https://www.health.harvard.edu/staying-healthy/exercise-and-aging-can-you-walk-away-from-father-time
- Fundazioa, E. F. (n.d.). *Study on 90-year-olds reveals the benefits of strength training.* Science Daily. Retrieved from https://www.sciencedaily.com/releases/2013/09/130927092350.htm

- Phillips, Stokes, Mcleod, J. M. T. S. S. P. (n.d.). *Resistance Exercise Training as a Primary Countermeasure to Age-Related Chronic Disease.* Frontiers in Physiology. Retrieved from https://www.frontiersin.org/articles/10.3389/fphys.2019.00645/full

- Maren, Cadore, Eduardo, Dorgo, Sandor Izquierdo, Mikel, Kraemer, William, Peterson, Mark, Ryan, Eric D., F. M. C. E. D. S. I. M. K. W. P. M. R. E. (n.d.). *Resistance Training for Older Adults: Position Statement From the National Strength and Conditioning Association.* National Strength and Conditioning Association. Retrieved from https://journals.lww.com/nsca-jscr/Fulltext/2019/08000/Resistance_Training_for_Older_Adults__Position.1.aspxSome

- Stemen, J. S. (n.d.). *Strength Training vs. Conditioning.* State of Fitness. Retrieved from https://mystateoffitness.com/strength-training-vs-conditioning/

- Johnson, K. J. (n.d.). *What is Conditioning Training? – Highly Beneficial!* Full Affect Fitness. Retrieved May 21, 2022, from https://fullaffectfitness.com/what-is-conditioning-training/

- White, K. W. (1993, November 1). *How the Mind Ages.* Psychology Today. Retrieved June 24, 2022, from https://www.psychologytoday.com/us/articles/199311/how-the-mind-ages

- Centers for Disease Control and Prevention. (n.d.). *Heart Disease Facts.* CDC. Retrieved from https://www.cdc.gov/heartdisease/facts.htm

- AHA Journals. (n.d.). *Heart Disease and Stroke Statistics—2021 Update.* Retrieved from https://www.ahajournals.org/doi/10.1161/CIR.0000000000000950

Chapter 2

- Rising Muscle. (n.d.). *HOW DOES STRENGTH TRAINING BOOST YOUR FITNESS AND HEALTH.* Rising Muscle Fitness Media. Retrieved from https://risingmuscle.com/how-does-strength-training-boost-your-fitness-and-health/

- Harvard Medical School. (n.d.). *Walking, other exercise helps seniors stay mobile, independent.* Harvard Health Blog. Retrieved from https://www.health.harvard.edu/blog/walking-exercise-helps-seniors-stay-mobile-independent-201405287173

- Strength Ambassadors. (n.d.). *Strong at any age: busting myths about strength training for older adults.* Strength Ambassadors. Com. Retrieved from https://strengthambassadors.com/blog/strength-training-older-people-myth-busted/

- Rush. (n.d.). *The Truth Behind Age-Old Myths.* Rush Stories. Retrieved from https://www.rush.edu/news/truth-behind-age-old-myths

- Griffin, M. G. (n.d.). *Myths About Exercise and Older Adults.* Compass by WebMD. Retrieved from https://www.webmd.com/healthy-aging/features/exercise-older-adults

- Tweed, K. T. (n.d.). *6 Myths about Aging.* Jump Start by WebMD. Retrieved from https://www.webmd.com/fitness-exercise/guide/exercise-and-aging-myths
- Joseph, Smith, Turley, D. P. S. R. T. T. N. J. (n.d.). *Strength-Training Myths.* University of Rochester Medical Center. Retrieved from https://www.urmc.rochester.edu/encyclopedia/content.aspx?ContentTypeID=1&ContentID=1492
- Argiles, J. M., & Rueda, R. (2016, June 17). *Journal of the American Medical Directors Association.* Retrieved from https://www.jamda.com/article/S1525-8610%2816%2930113-X/fulltext
- Arhen, D. K., & Lohr, B. A. (2005, July 25). *PSYCHOSOCIAL FACTORS IN SPORTS INJURY REHABILITATION.* ScienceDirect. Retrieved from https://www.sciencedirect.com/science/article/abs/pii/S0278591905700521
- Bahr, R., & Engebretsen, L. (2009, 0 0). *Handbook of Sports Medicine and Science.* Google Books. Retrieved from https://books.google.co.ke/books?hl=en&lr=&id=YqyDrQ1nLbUC&oi=fnd&pg=PT8&dq=sports+medicine+injury+prevention&ots=D-jDeXG0z1&sig=PMfRyczI_uNKvEVa4uVrcqZMB5I&redir_esc=y#v=onepage&q=sports%20medicine%20injury%20prevention&f=false
- Burr, D. B. (2002, April 29). *Effects of biomechanical stress on bones in animals - ScienceDirect.* Effects of Biomechanical Stress on Bones in Animals – ScienceDirect. Retrieved from https://www.sciencedirect.com/science/article/abs/pii/S875632820200707X
- Brukner et al. (2012). Brukner and Khan Clinical Sports Medicine. Google Books. Retrieved from FreeChapter.pdf (softtissuetherapyonline.com)
- *Can you boost your metabolism?: MedlinePlus Medical Encyclopedia.* (2020, May 26). Can You Boost Your Metabolism? MedlinePlus Medical Encyclopedia. Retrieved from https://medlineplus.gov/ency/patientinstructions/000893.htm
- Molé, P. A. (2012, October 7). *Impact of Energy Intake and Exercise on Resting Metabolic Rate - Sports Medicine.* SpringerLink; link.springer.com.https://link.springer.com/article/10.2165/00007256-199010020-00002
- *The Science Behind Strength Training to Burn Fat | Chuze Fitness.* (2015, March 31). Chuze Fitness; chuzefitness.com. https://chuzefitness.com/blog/science-strength-training-burn-fat/
- *Can you boost your metabolism?: MedlinePlus Medical Encyclopedia.* (2020, May 26). Can You Boost Your Metabolism?: MedlinePlus Medical Encyclopedia; medlineplus.gov.https://medlineplus.gov/ency/patientinstructions/000893.htm

- Waehner, P. (2020, June 17). *Beginner's Strength Training: How to Get Started.* Verywell Fit; www.verywellfit.com.https://www.verywellfit.com/complete-beginners-guide-to-strength-training-1229585
- Mountziaris, P. M., & Mikos, A. G. (2008, June 10). *Login to your account.* Liebertpub.Com; www.liebertpub.com.https://www.liebertpub.com/doi/abs/10.1089/ten.teb.2008.0038
- Burr, D. B. (2002, April 29). *Effects of biomechanical stress on bones in animals - ScienceDirect.* Effects of Biomechanical Stress on Bones in Animals - ScienceDirect; www.sciencedirect.com.https://www.sciencedirect.com/science/article/abs/pii/S875632820200707X
- *Exercise for Your Bone Health | NIH Osteoporosis and Related Bone Diseases National Resource Center.* (2018, October 1). Exercise for Your Bone Health | NIH Osteoporosis and Related Bone Diseases National Resource Center; www.bones.nih.gov.https://www.bones.nih.gov/health-info/bone/bone-health/exercise/exercise-your-bone-health
- Arhen, D. K., & Lohr, B. A. (2005, July 25). *PSYCHOSOCIAL FACTORS IN SPORTS INJURY REHABILITATION - ScienceDirect.* PSYCHOSOCIAL FACTORS IN SPORTS INJURY REHABILITATION - ScienceDirect; www.sciencedirect.com.https://www.sciencedirect.com/science/article/abs/pii/S0278591905700521
- Raglin, J. S. (2012, November 25). *Exercise and Mental Health - Sports Medicine.* SpringerLink; link.springer.com.https://link.springer.com/article/10.2165/00007256-199009060-00001
- Chang, C., Putukian, M., Aerni, G., Diamond, A., Hong, G., Ingram, Y., Reardon, C. L., & Wolanin, A. (2019, January 1). *Mental health issues and psychological factors in athletes: detection, management, effect on performance and prevention: American Medical Society for Sports Medicine Position Statement—Executive Summary.* British Journal of Sports Medicine. Retrieved May 21, 2022, fromhttps://bjsm.bmj.com/content/54/4/216.?int_source=trendmd&int_medium=cpc&int_campaign=usage-042019
- Chupel, M. U., Direito, F., Furtado, G. E., Minuzzi, L. G., Pedrosa, F. M., Colado, J. C., Ferreira, J. P., Filaire, E., & Teixeira, A. M. (2001, January 1). *Strength Training Decreases Inflammation and Increases Cognition and Physical Fitness in Older Women with Cognitive Impairment.* Frontiers. Retrieved fromhttps://www.frontiersin.org/articles/10.3389/fphys.2017.00377/full
- Claudino, J. G., Afonso, J., Sarvestan, J., Lanza, M. B., Pennone, J., Cardoso Filho, C. A., Serrão, J. C., Espregueira-Mendes, J., Vilefort Vasconcelos, A. L., de Andrade, M. P., Rocha-Rodrigues, S., Andrade, R., & Ramirez-Campillo, R. (2021, July 20). *JCM | Free Full-Text | Strength Training to Prevent Falls in Older Adults: A Systematic Review with Meta-Analysis of Randomized Controlled Trials.* Retrieved May 21, 2022, fromhttps://www.mdpi.com/2077-0383/10/14/3184

- *Exercise for Your Bone Health | NIH Osteoporosis and Related Bone Diseases National Resource Center.* (2018, October 1). Exercise for Your Bone Health | NIH Osteoporosis and Related Bone Diseases National Resource Center. Retrieved May 21, 2022, fromhttps://www.bones.nih.gov/health-info/bone/bone-health/exercise/exercise-your-bone-health
- Fentem, P. H. (1994, January 1). *ABC of Sports Medicine: Benefits of exercise in health and disease | The BMJ.* The BMJ. Retrieved from https://www.bmj.com/content/308/6939/1291.short
- Ferris, L. T., Williams, J. S., Shen, C. L., O'Keefe, K. A., & Hale, K. B. (2005, September 1). *Resistance Training Improves Sleep Quality in Older Adults a Pilot Study - PMC.* PubMed Central (PMC). Retrieved from https://www.ncbi.nlm.nih.gov/pmc/articles/PMC3887339/
- Gibala, M. J. (2012, November 29). *Protein Metabolism and Endurance Exercise - Sports Medicine.* SpringerLink. Retrieved May 21, 2022, fromhttps://link.springer.com/article/10.2165/00007256-200737040-00016
- Gordon, B. R., McDowell, C. P., Hallgren, M., Meyer, J. D., Lyons, M., & Herring, M. P. (2018, October 1). *Association of Resistance Exercise Training With Depressive Symptoms.* Association of Efficacy of Resistance Exercise Training With Depressive Symptoms: Meta-Analysis and Meta-Regression Analysis of Randomized Clinical Trials | Depressive Disorders | JAMA Psychiatry | JAMA Network. Retrieved May 21, 2022, fromhttps://jamanetwork.com/journals/jamapsychiatry/article-abstract/2680311
- Hansen, J. T. (2005). *Netter's Clinical Anatomy - John T. Hansen - Google Books.* Google Books. Retrieved fromhttps://books.google.co.ke/books?hl=en&lr=&id=RY5SEAAAQBAJ&oi=fnd&pg=PP1&dq=anatomy+by+netter&ots=HRYrOgtkpC&sig=xamtrEuYp5ne0BWitlqUqT-5Hpk&redir_esc=y#v=onepage&q=anatomy%20by%20netter&f=false
- *Healthy Muscles Matter: Ways to Care for the Muscular System.* (2017, March 9). National Institute of Arthritis and Musculoskeletal and Skin Diseases. Retrieved from https://www.niams.nih.gov/health-topics/kids/healthy-muscles
- *Increasing muscle strength can improve brain function: study - The University of Sydney.* (2016, October 25). The University of Sydney. Retrieved from https://www.sydney.edu.au/news-opinion/news/2016/10/25/increasing-muscle-strength-can-improve-brain-function--study.html
- Kell, R. T., Bell, G., & Quinney, A. (2012, November 13). *Musculoskeletal Fitness, Health Outcomes and Quality of Life - Sports Medicine.* SpringerLink. Retrieved from https://link.springer.com/article/10.2165/00007256-200131120-00003
- Lee, I.-H., & Park, S. (2014, January 8). *Balance Improvement by Strength Training for the Elderly - PMC.* PubMed Central (PMC). Retrieved from https://www.ncbi.nlm.nih.gov/pmc/articles/PMC3885846/

- L., S. K., & Suzzane, H. (2012, December 0). *Bone Health in Endurance Athletes: Runners, Cyclists, and...: Current Sports Medicine Reports.* LWW. Retrieved from https://journals.lww.com/acsm-csmr/Fulltext/2012/11000/Bone_Health_in_Endurance_Athletes__Runners,.14.aspx
- Messmer, D. (2022, April 19). *What Are Core Muscles? (with pictures).* The Health Board. Retrieved from https://www.thehealthboard.com/what-are-core-muscles.htm
- Molé, P. A. (2012, October 7). *Impact of Energy Intake and Exercise on Resting Metabolic Rate - Sports Medicine.* SpringerLink. Retrieved from https://link.springer.com/article/10.2165/00007256-199010020-00002
- Mountziaris, P. M., & Mikos, A. G. (2008, June 10). *Login to your account.* Liebertpub.Com. Retrieved from https://www.liebertpub.com/doi/abs/10.1089/ten.teb.2008.0038
- *Muscles: Types, composition, development, and more.* (2021, April 25). MedicalNewsToday. Retrieved from https://www.medicalnewstoday.com/articles/249192
- Paluska, S. A., & Schwenk, T. L. (2012, September 24). *Physical Activity and Mental Health - Sports Medicine.* SpringerLink. Retrieved from https://link.springer.com/article/10.2165/00007256-200029030-00003
- *Resistance training and functional plasticity of the aging brain: a 12-month randomized controlled trial.* (2011, July 7). Resistance Training and Functional Plasticity of the Aging Brain: A 12-Month Randomized Controlled Trial - ScienceDirect. Retrieved from https://www.sciencedirect.com/science/article/abs/pii/S019745801100193X
- Ricciotti, H. (2021, July 1). *Does exercise really boost energy levels? - Harvard Health.* Harvard Health. Retrieved from https://www.health.harvard.edu/exercise-and-fitness/does-exercise-really-boost-energy-levels
- Rodrigues, F., Domingos, C., Monteiro, D., & Morouço, P. (2022, January 13). *IJERPH | Free Full-Text | A Review on Aging, Sarcopenia, Falls, and Resistance Training in Community-Dwelling Older Adults.* Retrieved from https://www.mdpi.com/1660-4601/19/2/874/htm
- Raglin, J. S. (2012, November 25). *Exercise and Mental Health - Sports Medicine.* SpringerLink. Retrieved from https://link.springer.com/article/10.2165/00007256-199009060-00001
- Sadeghi, H., Shojaedin, S. S., Alijanpour, E., & Abbasi, A. (2020, April 1). *The Effects of Core Stability Exercises on Balance and Walking in Elderly Fallers with Mild Cognitive Impairment: A Randomized Control Trial.* The Effects of Core Stability Exercises on Balance and Walking in Elderly Fallers with Mild Cognitive Impairment: A Randomized Control Trial. Retrieved fromhttp://jrrs.mui.ac.ir/article_12838.html
- Silva-Batista, Carla1; de Brito, Leandro C.2; Corcos, Daniel M.3,4; Roschel, Hamilton1; de Mello, Marco T.5; Piemonte, Maria E.P.6; Tricoli, Valmor1; Ugrinowitsch, Carlos1 Resistance Training

Improves Sleep Quality in Subjects With Moderate Parkinson's Disease, Journal of Strength and Conditioning Research: August 2017 - Volume 31 - Issue 8 - p 2270-2277 doi: 10.1519/JSC.0000000000001685

- Shephard, R. J. (2012, September 30). *Sleep, Biorhythms and Human Performance - Sports Medicine.* SpringerLink. Retrieved from https://link.springer.com/article/10.2165/00007256-198401010-00003
- Stone, M., Plisk, S., & Collins, D. (2017, July 20). *Browse journals by subject.* Taylor& Francis Online. Retrieved from https://www.tandfonline.com/doi/abs/10.1080/14763140208522788
- *Strength and Conditioning for Grappling Sports: Strength & Conditioning Journal.* (2011, December 0). LWW. Retrieved from https://journals.lww.com/nsca-scj/fulltext/2011/12000/strength_and_conditioning_for_grappling_sports.4.aspx
- *Strength training and blood pressure - Harvard Health.* (2021, August 1). Harvard Health. Retrieved fromhttps://www.health.harvard.edu/heart-health/strength-training-and-blood-pressure
- *Strength Training for Stability and Mobility - Fort Wayne Pilates Classes.* (2021, July 16). Fort Wayne Pilates Classes. Retrieved fromhttps://puremovementstudio.com/2021/07/strength-training-for-stability-and-mobility/
- *Strength training could help you live longer, study finds.* (2018, August 28). The Independent. Retrieved from https://www.independent.co.uk/life-style/health-and-families/strength-training-muscle-stronger-live-longer-life-expectancy-increase-a8511491.html
- *The Science Behind Strength Training to Burn Fat | Chuze Fitness.* (2015, March 31). Chuze Fitness. Retrieved fromhttps://chuzefitness.com/blog/science-strength-training-burn-fat/
- *The Mental Health Benefits Of Strength Training | Psychology Today.* (2022, May 1). Psychology Today. Retrieved fromhttps://www.psychologytoday.com/us/blog/the-bonds-we-make/201807/the-mental-health-benefits-strength-training
- Training, T. T. (2021, September 21). *How Does Strength Training Help Balance and Improve Hormone Levels? - Top Tyr Training.* Top Tyr Training. Retrieved from https://www.toptyrtraining.com/how-does-strength-training-help-balance-and-improve-hormone-levels/
- Tortora, G. J., & Derrickson, B. (2016, October 27). Google Books. Retrieved from https://books.google.co.ke/books?hl=en&lr=&id=aSaVDwAAQBAJ&oi=fnd&pg=PR4&dq=principles+of+anatomy+and+physiology+by+tortora&ots=le3mWI2BsN&sig=ZhwogaU5MQVodQ-V680xNROZesw&redir_esc=y#v=onepage&q=principles%20of%20anatomy%20and%20physiology%20by%20tortora&f=false
- Vranish, J. R., & Bailey, E. F. (2016, June 1). *Inspiratory Muscle Training Improves Sleep and Mitigates Cardiovascular Dysfunction in Obstructive Sleep Apnea | SLEEP | Oxford Academic.* OUP Academic. Retrieved from https://academic.oup.com/sleep/article/39/6/1179/2453931?login=true

- Waehner, P. (2020, June 17). *Beginner's Strength Training: How to Get Started.* Verywell Fit. Retrieved from https://www.verywellfit.com/complete-beginners-guide-to-strength-training-1229585
- Walden, M. (2016, October 20). *Core Muscles & Benefits of Core Stability Explained.* Sportsinjuryclinic. Retrieved fromhttps://www.sportsinjuryclinic.net/rehabilitation-exercises/core-strengthening-exercises/introduction-to-core-strengthening
- Watson, Andrew M. MD, MS Sleep and Athletic Performance, Current Sports Medicine Reports: 11/12 2017 - Volume 16 - Issue 6 - p 413-418 doi: 10.1249/JSR.0000000000000418
- Westcott, Wayne L. Ph.D. Resistance Training is Medicine, Current Sports Medicine Reports: July/August 2012 - Volume 11 - Issue 4 - p 209-216 doi: 10.1249/JSR.0b013e31825dabb8
- *Weight training may boost brain power - Harvard Health.* (2017, January 1). Harvard Health. Retrieved fromhttps://www.health.harvard.edu/mind-and-mood/weight-training-may-boost-brain-power
- *What is Strength & Conditioning? - Strength and Conditioning Education.* (2019, August 30). Strength and Conditioning Education. Retrieved May 21, 2022, fromhttps://strengthandconditioningeducation.com/what-is-strength-conditioning/#:~:text=%20What%20are%20the%20benefits%20of%20strength%20and,truth%20universally%20acknowledged%20that%20exercise%20is...%20More%20
- *What You Need to Know About Hormone Therapy for Improving Memory.* (2017, August 8). Balance Hormone Center. Retrieved from https://www.balancehormonecenter.com/blog/hormone-therapy-for-improving-memory/
- *Why Is the Muscular System so Important?* (2015, August 4). Reference.Com. Retrieved fromhttps://www.reference.com/science/muscular-system-important-570e88dd98b54386

Chapter 3

- Lifestyle, L. (n.d.). *12 Tips On How To Start Something New.* Believe in Help. Retrieved from https://believeinhelp.com/12-tips-on-how-to-start-something-new/
- Briggs, S. B. (n.d.). *25 Ways to Develop a Growth Mindset.* InformED. Retrieved from https://www.opencolleges.edu.au/informed/features/develop-a-growth-mindset/
- Cherry, K. C. (n.d.). *What Is a Mindset and Why It Matters.* Very Well Mind. Retrieved from, S. L. (n.d.). *What is Motivation? Why It is Important and How to Get It.* Stunning Motivation. Retrieved from https://www.verywellmind.com/what-is-a-mindset-2795025
- Lim, S. L. (n.d.). *What is Motivation? Why It is Important and How to Get It.* Stunning Motivation. Retrieved from https://stunningmotivation.com/what-is-motivation/

- Vanbuskirk, S. V. (n.d.). *How to Get Motivated: Tips to Help You Find Motivation.* Goalcast. Retrieved from https://www.goalcast.com/how-to-get-motivated/
- Copeland, B. C. (n.d.). *SMART Goals How to Make Your Goals Achievable.* Mind Tools. Retrieved from https://www.mindtools.com/pages/article/smart-goals.htm
- Lim, S. L. (n.d.). *13 Ways How to Celebrate Small Victories and Make Progress.* Stunning Motivation. Retrieved from https://stunningmotivation.com/celebrate-small-victories/
- *Form Good Habits.* (n.d.). Content Byui.Edu. Retrieved from https://content.byui.edu/file/b8b83119-9acc-4a7b-bc84-efacf9043998/1/Learning-1-2-2.html
- Savov, P. S. (n.d.). *Why Have a Coach - 15 Great Benefits of Coaching.* Noomi, The Professional Coaching Directory. Retrieved from https://www.noomii.com/articles/12518-why-have-a-coach-15-great-benefits-of-coaching
- Chadwick, S. C. (n.d.). *5 Benefits of Accountability.* Accountable to You. Retrieved from https://accountable2you.com/blog/benefits-of-accountability/
- Augustyn, A. A. (n.d.). *Mario Lemieux.* Britannica. Retrieved June 11, 2022, from https://www.britannica.com/biography/Mario-Lemieux
- Wikimedia Foundation. (n.d.). *Mario Lemieux.* Wikipedia, The Free Encyclopedia. Retrieved June 11, 2022, from https://en.wikipedia.org/wiki/Mario_Lemieux
- Human Kinetics - An Employee Owned Company. (n.d.). *THE THREE COMPONENTS OF MOTIVATION AFFECT EXERCISE ADHERENCE.* Human Kinetics. Retrieved June 11, 2022, from https://us.humankinetics.com/blogs/excerpt/the-three-components-of-motivation-affect-exercise-adherence
- IPL, I. P. L. (n.d.). *Three Components Of Motivation.* Ipl. Retrieved June 11, 2022, from https://www.ipl.org/essay/Three-Components-Of-Motivation-FCKCE65YZNR
- Taylor, J. T. (n.d.). *Sports: What Motivates Athletes?* Psychology Today. Retrieved June 11, 2022, from https://www.psychologytoday.com/us/blog/the-power-prime/200910/sports-what-motivates-athletes
- Locke, R. L. (n.d.). *The Stories Of These 5 Athletes Will Motivate Everyone Of You.* Lifehack. Retrieved June 11, 2022, from https://www.lifehack.org/articles/communication/the-stories-these-5-athletes-will-motivate-everyone-you.html
- Dawson, C. D. (n.d.). *How being realistic can be key to your wellbeing.* BBC. Retrieved June 11, 2022, from https://www.bbc.com/worklife/article/20200722-how-being-realistic-can-be-key-to-your-wellbeing
- Chowdhury, M. R. C. (n.d.). *The Science & Psychology Of Goal-Setting 101.* Positive Psychology. Retrieved June 11, 2022, from https://positivepsychology.com/goal-setting-psychology/#:~:text=The%20Psychology%20Of%20Goal%20Setting,-

Goals%20play%20a&text=Studies%20have%20shown%20that%20when,essential%20part%20of%20our%20identity

- Bradshaw, H. B. (2021, May 12). *Elon Musk's Mindset Key to Accelerate Success.* Medium. Retrieved June 26, 2022, from https://medium.com/illumination/elon-musks-mindset-key-to-accelerate-success-6392f67bf3d
- https://populartimelines.com/timeline/Elon-Musk
- https://financhill.com/blog/investing/how-did-elon-musk-make-his-money

Chapter 4

- Chowdhury, M. R. C. (2019, May 2). *The Science & Psychology Of Goal-Setting 101.* Positive Psychology. Retrieved June 14, 2022, from https://positivepsychology.com/goal-setting-psychology/#:~:text=Arends%2C%20201
- Goodman, N. G. (n.d.). *The Science of Setting Goals.* Ideas TED. Retrieved June 11, 2022, from https://ideas.ted.com/the-science-of-setting-goals/
- Locke, Latham, E. L. G. L. (n.d.). *Building a Practically Useful Theory of Goal Setting and Task Motivation: A 35Year Odyssey.* Research Gate. Retrieved June 11, 2022, from https://www.researchgate.net/publication/254734316_Building_a_Practically_Useful_Theory_of_Goal_Setting_and_Task_Motivation_A_35Year_Odyssey
- *The 10 Fitness Goals You Should Be Setting.* (n.d.). Runner's Blueprint. Retrieved June 11, 2022, from https://www.runnersblueprint.com/fitness-goals/
- Kenyon, Z. K. (2015, March 31). *11 of J.K. Rowling's most inspiring quotes on failure.* Cosmopolitan. Retrieved June 14, 2022, from https://www.cosmopolitan.com/uk/entertainment/a34577/jk-rowling-inspiring-quotes-failure-imagination/
- *Steve Jobs' dent in the universe—the shocking truth revealed!* (n.d.). Solve Next. Retrieved June 14, 2022, from https://solvenext.com/blog/steve-jobs-dent-in-the-universethe-shocking-truth-revealed
- Murphy, M. M. (2015, January 8). *"SMART" Goals Can Sometimes Be Dumb.* Forbes. Retrieved June 14, 2022, from https://www.forbes.com/sites/markmurphy/2015/01/08/smart-goals-can-sometimes-be-dumb/?sh=107037d1718e
- Pandey, D. P. (2017, January 17). *Why You Shouldn't Be Afraid to Set Irrational Goals.* Fortune. Retrieved June 14, 2022, from https://fortune.com/2017/06/07/goal-setting-entrepreneurs-amazon-apple/
- Dykstra, J. D. (2019, October 16). *HERE'S HOW MUCH MONEY BRUCE LEE WAS WORTH WHEN HE DIED. Read More: https://www.grunge.com/170282/heres-how-much-money-bruce-lee-was-worth-when-he-died/?utm_campaign=clip.* Grunge. Retrieved June 14, 2022, from https://www.grunge.com/170282/heres-how-much-money-bruce-lee-was-worth-when-he-died/

- University of Georgia. (n.d.). *SMART GOALS*. Retrieved June 14, 2022, from https://open.online.uga.edu/fitness/chapter/smartgoals/
- Fox, J. F. (2020, July 24). *How To Set SMART Fitness Goals*. Nutrioneering. Retrieved June 14, 2022, from https://www.bodybuildingmealplan.com/smart-fitness-goals/
- Vanbuskirk, S. V. (n.d.). *SMART Fitness Goals Examples to Motivate You*. Goalcast. Retrieved June 14, 2022, from https://www.goalcast.com/smart-fitness-goals-examples/
- Mind Tools Content Team. (n.d.). *SMART Goals How to Make Your Goals Achievable*. Mind Tools. Retrieved June 14, 2022, from https://www.mindtools.com/pages/article/smart-goals.htm

Chapter 5

- Davidson, K. D. (n.d.). *How Can You Maintain a Healthy Diet?* Healthline. Retrieved June 11, 2022, from https://www.healthline.com/health/healthy-eating-for-seniors#healthy-diet
- Spraul, T. S. (n.d.). *WHY IS NUTRITION IMPORTANT WHEN EXERCISING?* Exercise.Com. Retrieved June 11, 2022, from https://www.exercise.com/learn/why-is-nutrition-important-when-exercising/
- Ellis, E. E. (n.d.). *Healthy Eating for Older Adults*. Eat Right. Retrieved June 11, 2022, from https://www.eatright.org/food/nutrition/dietary-guidelines-and-myplate/healthy-eating-for-older-adults
- Graham, J. G., & The Washington Post. (2019, January 19). *For older adults, a protein-rich diet is important for health*. The Washington Post. Retrieved June 15, 2022, from https://www.washingtonpost.com/national/health-science/for-older-adults-a-protein-rich-diet-is-important-for-health/2019/01/18/886926ce-1a78-11e9-88fe-f9f77a3bcb6c_story.html
- McManus, K. D. M. (2019, June 20). *Healthy eating for older adults*. Harvard Health Publishing. Retrieved July 8, 2022, from https://www.health.harvard.edu/blog/healthy-eating-for-older-adults-2019062016868
- *Protein Quality Matters*. (n.d.). ProPortion Foods. Retrieved June 11, 2022, from https://www.proportionfoods.com.au/protein-quality-matters/#:~:text=Protein%20quality%20can%20be%20simply,consumption%20%5B3%2C4%5D
- Broxterman, J. B. (n.d.). *Nutrition for seniors: 7 lifestyle strategies to stay strong, healthy, and independent longer*. Precision Nutrition. Retrieved June 14, 2022, from https://www.precisionnutrition.com/nutrition-for-seniors
- Micu, A. M. (2018, April 23). *Proper hydration helps seniors get the full benefit of exercise and keeps their minds limber*. ZME Science. Retrieved June 14, 2022, from https://www.zmescience.com/science/seniors-exercise-water-243422/

- Jones, E. B. J. (2022, May 15). *Adult Dehydration.* National Library of Medicine. Retrieved June 14, 2022, from https://www.ncbi.nlm.nih.gov/books/NBK555956/
- National Council of Aging. (2021, August 8). *How to Stay Hydrated for Better Health.* Retrieved June 14, 2022, from https://www.ncoa.org/article/how-to-stay-hydrated-for-better-health
- Iora with one medical. (2021, July 15). *Best Protein-Rich Foods for Seniors.* Retrieved June 14, 2022, from https://ioraprimarycare.com/blog/best-protein-rich-foods-for-seniors/
- Baum, Kim, Wolfe, J. B. Y. K. W. F. (2016, June 8). *Protein Consumption and the Elderly: What Is the Optimal Level of Intake?* National Library of Medicine. Retrieved June 14, 2022, from https://www.ncbi.nlm.nih.gov/pmc/articles/PMC4924200/
- Dodd, K. D. (202–08-29). *Protein Requirements for Older Adults.* The Geriatric Dietitian. Retrieved June 14, 2022, from https://thegeriatricdietitian.com/protein-requirements-for-older-adults/
- Kaselj, R. K. (2017, November 14). *Pros & Cons of Different Types of Sugar.* Exercises for Injuries. Retrieved June 14, 2022, from https://exercisesforinjuries.com/pros-cons-different-types-sugar/
- Yes Health. (2021, November 23). *Whole Foods vs. Processed Foods.* Yes Health. Retrieved June 14, 2022, from https://blog.yeshealth.com/consumer/whole-foods-vs.-processed-foods
- Harvard Health Publishing. (2022, January 6). *The sweet danger of sugar.* Harvard Health. Retrieved June 14, 2022, from https://www.health.harvard.edu/heart-health/the-sweet-danger-of-sugar
- Lustig, Schmidt, Brindis, R. L. S. C. B. (2014, February 1). *The toxic truth about sugar.* Nature. Retrieved June 14, 2022, from https://www.nature.com/articles/482027a
- Basu, D. B. B. (2021, October 10). *Pros and Cons of Consuming Sugar.* Author DB Basu. Retrieved June 14, 2022, from https://bdbasu.com/pros-and-cons-of-consuming-sugar/
- Dr. Health Benefits. (n.d.). *10 Benefits of Sugar for Health.* Dr. Health Benefits. Retrieved June 14, 2022, from https://drhealthbenefits.com/food-bevarages/flavourings/benefits-sugar-health
- Hill, L. H. (2021, April 22). *Breakfast: Is It the Most Important Meal?* WebMD. Retrieved June 14, 2022, from https://www.webmd.com/food-recipes/breakfast-lose-weight
- Spence, C. S. (2017, July). *Breakfast: The most important meal of the day?* Science Direct. Retrieved June 14, 2022, from https://www.sciencedirect.com/science/article/pii/S1878450X17300045
- *Nutritional Update for Physicians: Plant-Based Diets.* (n.d.). The National Library of Medicine. Retrieved June 14, 2022, from https://www.ncbi.nlm.nih.gov/pmc/articles/PMC3662288/
- National University of Natural Medicine. (n.d.). *Plant-Based Diets: Pros and Cons According to NUNM.* Retrieved June 14, 2022, from https://nunm.edu/2019/04/plant-based-diets/
- Healthline. (n.d.). 26 Muscle Building Foods to Add to Your Diet. Healthline. Retrieved June 14, 2022, from https://www.healthline.com/nutrition/26-muscle-building-foods#TOC_TITLE_HDR_6

- Weishaupt, J. W. (2021, November 24). What Are Plant Food Sources of Vitamin B12? WebMD. Retrieved July 8, 2022, from https://www.webmd.com/diet/what-are-plant-food-sources-vitamin-b12

Chapter 6

- *3 Easy Ways to Prepare Your Body for a Hard Workout - wikiHow.* (2021, May 31). Retrieved May 28, 2022, fromhttps://www.wikihow.com/Prepare-Your-Body-for-a-Hard-Workout
- *8 Ways to Reduce Lactic Acid Build-Up From Exercising - Weight Belt Fitness.* (2019, November 21). Weight Belt Fitness. Retrieved May 28, 2022, from https://www.weightbeltfitness.com/8-ways-to-reduce-lactic-acid-build-up-from-exercising/
- Andrews, R. (2010, January 11). *All About Post-Workout Nutrition - Precision Nutrition.* Precision Nutrition. Retrieved May 28, 2022, from https://www.precisionnutrition.com/about-post-workout-nutrition
- Areta, J. L., & Hopkins, W. G. (2018). Skeletal muscle glycogen content at rest and during endurance exercise in humans: a meta-analysis. *Sports Medicine, 48*(9), 2091-2102.
- Bajwa, A. (2022, March 29). *How To Stretch Correctly.* Scoopearth.Com. Retrieved May 28, 2022, fromhttps://www.scoopearth.com/how-to-stretch-correctly/
- Bartlett, M. J., & Warren, P. J. (n.d.). *Effect of warming up on knee proprioception before sporting activity.* British Journal of Sports Medicine; bjsm.bmj.com. Retrieved May 29, 2022, fromhttps://bjsm.bmj.com/content/36/2/132.short
- Bonvenchio, T. (2020, August 24). *The Do's and Don'ts of Stretching As a Warmup | Fitness | MyFitnessPal.* MyFitnessPal Blog. Retrieved May 28, 2022, fromhttps://blog.myfitnesspal.com/the-dos-and-donts-of-stretching-as-a-warmup/
- Brotherhood, J. R. (1984). Nutrition and sports performance. *Sports Medicine, 1*(5), 350-389.
- Brouns, F., Rehrer, N. J., M. Saris, W. H., Beckers, E., Menheere, P., & Hoor, F. ten. (2008, March 14). *Thieme E-Journals - International Journal of Sports Medicine / Abstract.* Thieme E-Journals - International Journal of Sports Medicine / Abstract. Retrieved May 29, 2022, fromhttps://www.thieme-connect.com/products/ejournals/abstract/10.1055/s-2007-1024956
- Bucci, L. R. (2020). *Nutrition applied to injury rehabilitation and sports medicine.* CRC Press.
- Catanzaro, J. P. (2014, September 23). *How To Stretch Properly: The Do's And Don'ts Of Stretching.* Bodybuilding.Com. Retrieved May 28, 2022, fromhttps://www.bodybuilding.com/content/how-to-stretch-properly-the-dos-and-donts-of-stretching.html
- Cerin. (2009, October 5). *Warming up – Do's and don'ts of a general warm-up. - Rees Fitness.* Retrieved May 28, 2022, fromhttps://reesfitness.co.uk/blog/2009/10/05/warming-up-dos-and-donts-of-a-general-warm-up/

- CES, PES, J. B. (2017, August 14). *How To Get Enough Post Workout Sleep For Maximum Results - Fitneass.* Fitneass. Retrieved May 28, 2022, from https://www.fitneass.com/post-workout-sleep/
- Fradkin, A. J., & Gabbe, B. J. (2006, May 6). *Does warming up prevent injury in sport?: The evidence from randomised controlled trials?* Does Warming up Prevent Injury in Sport?: The Evidence from Randomised Controlled Trials? - ScienceDirect. Retrieved May 29, 2022, fromhttps://www.sciencedirect.com/science/article/abs/pii/S144024400600051X
- Fradkin, Andrea J1; Zazryn, Tsharni R2; Smoliga, James M3 Effects of Warming-up on Physical Performance: A Systematic Review With Meta-analysis, Journal of Strength and Conditioning Research: January 2010 - Volume 24 - Issue 1 - p 140-148 doi: 10.1519/JSC.0b013e3181c643a0
- Freitas de Salles, B., Simao, R., Miranda, F., da Silva Novaes, J., Lemos, A., & Willardson, J. M. (2009). Rest interval between sets in strength training. *Sports medicine*, *39*(9), 765-777.
- Friedrich, C. (2018, February 4). *Do You Really Need More Exercise Recovery Time as You Age?* Cathe Friedrich. Retrieved May 28, 2022, fromhttps://cathe.com/really-need-exercise-recovery-time-age/
- Gibson, S., Nigrovic, L. E., O'Brien, M., & Meehan III, W. P. (2013). The effect of recommending cognitive rest on recovery from sport-related concussion. *Brain injury*, *27*(7-8), 839-842.
- Gil, Maria Helena MD1,2; Neiva, Henrique P. PhD1,2; Sousa, António C. MD1,2; Marques, Mário C. PhD1,2; Marinho, Daniel A. PhD1,2 Current Approaches on Warming up for Sports Performance: A Critical Review, Strength and Conditioning Journal: August 2019 - Volume 41 - Issue 4 - p 70-79 doi: 10.1519/SSC.0000000000000454
- Hawley, J. A., & Leckey, J. J. (2015). Carbohydrate dependence during prolonged, intense endurance exercise. *Sports Medicine*, *45*(1), 5-12.
- *How to Prepare Your Body for a Workout - The Monday Campaigns.* (2022, January 10). The Monday Campaigns. Retrieved May 28, 2022, fromhttps://www.mondaycampaigns.org/move-it-monday/how-to-prepare-your-body-for-a-workout
- Kedia, A. W., Hofheins, J. E., Habowski, S. M., Ferrando, A. A., Gothard, M. D., & Lopez, H. L. (2014, January 2). *Effects of a Pre-workout Supplement on Lean Mass, Muscular Performance, Subjective Workout Experience and Biomarkers of Safety - PMC.* PubMed Central (PMC). Retrieved May 29, 2022, fromhttps://www.ncbi.nlm.nih.gov/pmc/articles/PMC3894395/
- Madbarz. (2015, November 10). *Warm Up: Do's and Don'ts.* Madbarz. Retrieved May 28, 2022, fromhttps://www.madbarz.com/blog/101-warm-up-dos-and-donts
- Marson, G. (2021, July 21). *The Benefits of Visualization - Power of Visualization - Dr. Gia Marson.* Gia Marson. Retrieved May 28, 2022, fromhttps://drgiamarson.com/the-benefits-of-visualization/#:~:text=%20When%20done%20right%2C%20a%20regular%20visualization%20practice,Improve%20mood%2014%20Declutter%20your%20mind%20More%20

- Parcell, A. C., Sawyer, R. D., Tricoli, V. A., & Chinevere, T. D. (2002). Minimum rest period for strength recovery during a common isokinetic testing protocol. *Medicine and science in sports and exercise, 34*(6), 1018-1022.
- Preuss, S. (2022, March 21). *How to Breathe Properly During Your Workout.* The Perfect Workout. Retrieved May 28, 2022, fromhttps://www.theperfectworkout.com/breathe-properly-during-workout/
- Quaglio, L. (n.d.). *The Right Way to Breathe During Exercise.* The Right Way to Breathe During Exercise; blog.nasm.org. Retrieved May 28, 2022, fromhttps://blog.nasm.org/the-right-way-to-breathe-during-exercise
- Rodriguez, N. R., Di Marco, N. M., & Langley, S. (2009). American College of Sports Medicine position stand. Nutrition and athletic performance. *Medicine and science in sports and exercise, 41*(3), 709-731.
- Rusin, T Nation, D. J., Rusin, D. J., Ph.D., J. S., Murphy, D., Ph.D., D. L., & Somerset, D. (2015, February 11). *The Most Intelligent Way to Warm Up.* T NATION. Retrieved May 28, 2022, fromhttps://www.t-nation.com/training/the-most-intelligent-way-to-warm-up/
- Semeco, A. (2018, May 31). *Pre-Workout Nutrition: What to Eat Before a Workout.* Healthline. Retrieved May 28, 2022, fromhttps://www.healthline.com/nutrition/eat-before-workout#TOC_TITLE_HDR_2
- Shellock, F. G., & Prentice, W. E. (2012, December 11). *Warming-Up and Stretching for Improved Physical Performance and Prevention of Sports-Related Injuries - Sports Medicine.* SpringerLink. Retrieved May 29, 2022, fromhttps://link.springer.com/article/10.2165/00007256-198502040-00004
- Thomas, D. T., Erdman, K. A., & Burke, L. M. (2016). American College of Sports Medicine Joint Position Statement. Nutrition and Athletic Performance. *Medicine and science in sports and exercise, 48*(3), 543-568.
- Vitale, K. C., Owens, R., Hopkins, S. R., & Malhotra, A. (2019). Sleep hygiene for optimizing recovery in athletes: review and recommendations. *International journal of sports medicine, 40*(08), 535-543.
- Voropay, E. (2015, April 15). *Visualization Techniques - Mental Tips for Better Workouts.* ShapeFit.Com. Retrieved May 28, 2022, fromhttps://www.shapefit.com/exercise/visualization-techniques-workouts.html
- *Warm-Up Dos and Don'ts - Fit People.* (2019, January 12). Fit People. Retrieved May 28, 2022, fromhttps://fitpeople.com/fitness/warm-up-dos-and-donts/
- Watson, A. M. (2017). Sleep and athletic performance. *Current sports medicine reports, 16*(6), 413-418.
- *Why is hydration important during exercise?.* (n.d.). Hydrant. Retrieved May 28, 2022, fromhttps://www.drinkhydrant.com/blogs/news/hydration-and-exercise

- Wiktorsson-Moller M, Öberg B, Ekstrand J, Gillquist J. Effects of warming up, massage, and stretching on range of motion and muscle strength in the lower extremity. The American Journal of Sports Medicine. 1983;11(4):249-252. doi:10.1177/036354658301100412
- Layden, T. L. (2010, February 17). *Ready to Rock*. Sports Illustrated. Retrieved June 22, 2022, from https://www.si.com/more-sports/2010/02/17/vonn
- **Chapter 7**
- Lindberg, S. L. (2022, January 22). *9 Chair Exercises That Will Light Up Your Entire Body*. SELF. Retrieved June 22, 2022, from https://www.self.com/gallery/chair-exercises
- Graves, W. G. (2020, June 23). *Do you Need an Exercise Mat?* Fabrication Enterprises Inc. Retrieved June 22, 2022, from https://www.fab-ent.com/do-you-need-an-exercise-mat/#:~:text=Exercise%20mats%20can%20help%20stabilize,are%20preferred%20by%20many%20people
- The Turkish Towel Company. (2019, May 19). *HOW TO CHOOSE THE PERFECT GYM TOWEL*. The Turkish Towel Company. Retrieved June 22, 2022, from https://turkishtowelcompany.com/how-to-choose-the-perfect-gym-towel/#:~:text=Gym%20towels%20are%20so%20important,with%20bacteria%20on%20gym%20equipment
- Mendoza, M. F. M. (2021, September 4). *Surprising benefits of lifting light weights at home Read more: https://lifestyle.inquirer.net/389223/surprising-benefits-of-lifting-light-weights-at-home/#ixzz7WvAR37sO Follow us: @inquirerdotnet on Twitter | inquirerdotnet on Facebook*. Lifestyle.INQ. Retrieved June 22, 2022, from https://lifestyle.inquirer.net/389223/surprising-benefits-of-lifting-light-weights-at-home/
- Health Essentials. (2022, May 4). *How Effective Are Resistance Bands for Strength Training?* Cleaveland Clinic. Retrieved June 22, 2022, from https://health.clevelandclinic.org/should-you-try-resistance-bands-for-strength-training/
- **Chapter 8**
- Lambkin, M. L. (n.d.). *As a Beginner, How Long Should You WorkOut?* Planet Fitness. Retrieved June 22, 2022, from https://www.planetfitness.com/community/articles/beginner-how-long-should-i-work-out#:~:text=Try%20starting%20with%20short%20workouts,%2Dtraining%20sessions%2C%20per%20week
- Shepherd, B. S. (2022, May). *What is progressive overload?* Live Science. Retrieved June 22, 2022, from https://www.livescience.com/what-is-progressive-overload
- Salyer, J. S. (2016, April 4). *What Is Progressive Overload Training?* Healthline. Retrieved June 22, 2022, from https://www.healthline.com/health/progressive-overload#examples

- Adams, A. A. (n.d.). *PROGRESSIVE OVERLOAD EXPLAINED: GROW MUSCLE & STRENGTH TODAY*. NASM. Retrieved June 22, 2022, from https://blog.nasm.org/progressive-overload-explained
- MasterClass Staff. (2022, February 24). *Progressive Overload: 6 Progressive Overload Techniques*. Master Class. Retrieved June 22, 2022, from https://www.masterclass.com/articles/progressive-overload-guide

Made in the USA
Las Vegas, NV
20 February 2023

67847419R00103